BEHAVIORAL AND PSYCHOLOGICAL
SYMPTOMS OF DEMENTIA

BEHAVIORAL AND PSYCHOLOGICAL
SYMPTOMS OF DEMENTIA

Art Walaszek, M.D.

Professor, Vice Chair for Education and Faculty Development,
Residency Training Director, Department of Psychiatry
Co-Leader, Outreach, Recruitment and Education Core,
Wisconsin Alzheimer's Disease Research Center
Public Health Pillar Leader, Wisconsin Alzheimer's Institute
University of Wisconsin School of Medicine and Public Health, Madison

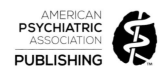

AMERICAN
PSYCHIATRIC
ASSOCIATION
PUBLISHING

Note: The author has worked to ensure that all information in this book is accurate at the time of publication and consistent with general psychiatric and medical standards, and that information concerning drug dosages, schedules, and routes of administration is accurate at the time of publication and consistent with standards set by the U.S. Food and Drug Administration and the general medical community. As medical research and practice continue to advance, however, therapeutic standards may change. Moreover, specific situations may require a specific therapeutic response not included in this book. For these reasons and because human and mechanical errors sometimes occur, we recommend that readers follow the advice of physicians directly involved in their care or the care of a member of their family.

Books published by American Psychiatric Association Publishing represent the findings, conclusions, and views of the individual authors and do not necessarily represent the policies and opinions of American Psychiatric Association Publishing or the American Psychiatric Association.

The author acknowledges receipt of *honoraria* from the Wisconsin Association of Medical Directors to lecture on the topic of behavioral and psychological symptoms of dementia, the Advocate Lutheran General Hospital, and United Way/Pharmacy Society of Wisconsin; *grant support* from National Institute on Aging, U.S. Administration on Community Living, and UW Wisconsin Partnership Program; *advance on royalties* from American Psychiatric Association Publishing; and as *investigator* (not compensated) for Eisai Network Companies.

If you wish to buy 50 or more copies of the same title, please go to www.appi.org/specialdiscounts for more information.

Library of Congress Cataloging-in-Publication Data
Names: Walaszek, Art, 1972– author. | American Psychiatric Association
    Publishing, publisher.
Title: Behavioral and psychological symptoms of dementia / Art Walaszek.
Description: Washington, D.C. : American Psychiatric Association Publishing,
    [2020] | Includes bibliographical references and index.
Identifiers: LCCN 2019018640 (print) | LCCN 2019019219 (ebook) | ISBN
    9781615372676 (ebook) | ISBN 9781615371686 (pbk. : alk. paper)
Subjects: | MESH: Alzheimer Disease—diagnosis | Alzheimer Disease—therapy |
    Neurobehavioral Manifestations | Symptom Assessment
Classification: LCC RC523 (ebook) | LCC RC523 (print) | NLM WT 155 | DDC
    616.8/311—dc23
LC record available at https://lccn.loc.gov/2019018640

British Library Cataloguing in Publication Data
A CIP record is available from the British Library.

Contents

FOREWORD

More than 5 million people in the United States have Alzheimer's dementia, and by 2050 the number is expected to rise to nearly 14 million (Alzheimer's Association 2018). In 2018, Alzheimer's disease was the sixth leading cause of death (Alzheimer's Association 2018), and many millions of family members and other informal caregivers provide the care necessary for many people with Alzheimer's and other dementias to live in the community. Additionally, the number of people entering geriatric psychiatry and geriatric medicine specialty fellowships and practices has been declining relative to the increase in the number of older adults in the United States (Bragg et al. 2010, 2012). Institute of Medicine committees examining the workforce for geriatric medicine and for geriatric mental health and substance use both concluded that the United States will be woefully short of having enough specialists to meet the needs of the growing elderly population (Institute of Medicine 2008, 2012). Therefore, Dr. Walaszek's book *Behavioral and Psychological Symptoms of Dementia* is timely and greatly needed, because its aim is to help primary care providers address behavioral and psychological symptoms of dementia, some of the most common problems that would cause patients to otherwise be referred for geriatric psychiatry care.

In this concise but comprehensive book, Dr. Walaszek covers the full range of behavioral and psychological symptoms of dementia encountered by patients and their families and primary care providers, while also providing the necessary foundations to distinguish the different types of dementia, the key elements of patient history needed to develop an appropriate treatment approach, and the basic medical and laboratory workups that should be performed. Each chapter begins with a brief précis; well-written descriptions of the major topic follow; and key points summarize the chapter's content. The chapters cover the common types of behavioral and emotional symptoms as well as the important associated system issues relevant to dementia care, including elder abuse reporting, creating advance directives and power of attorney arrangements, safety planning, and caregiver support resources.

Dr. Walaszek provides an up-to-date review of the literature that strikes an appropriate balance in clarifying new and promising findings that are being developed but that are not yet applicable to current standard-of-care practices. Similarly, the book readily acknowledges where there are significant gaps in the literature. Standard-of-care pharmacological and psychosocial approaches in the management of behavioral and psychological symptoms of dementia are presented with a realistic understanding of the benefits and difficulties of providing each treatment. Relevant information on complementary medicine is included, and the book covers personality, cultural, and spiritual domains so that one is always reminded of the whole-person approach in delivering this care. To provide a practical interpretation of how to incorporate research findings and established standard-of-care practices, Dr. Walaszek often informs the reader of precisely how he manages aspects of care in his own practice. He describes patient scenarios that are common across clinical settings from outpatient, hospital, and nursing home locations.

Although the book is written principally for primary care providers, the extensive literature review that Dr. Walaszek provides also makes the book useful for general practice psychiatrists who have not stayed as up to date on the geriatric psychiatry literature. His many years of experience and dedication to resident education are evident in the book's clear organization and his succinct writing. Therefore, even those in academia who specialize in geriatric medicine or psychiatry will find the book useful for organizing and teaching this material to students, residents, and fellows. The book is a welcome addition to the growing literature on geriatric psychiatry and dementia care in particular.

Mark Snowden, M.D., M.P.H.
Associate Professor
Psychiatry and Behavioral Sciences
University of Washington School of Medicine, Seattle

REFERENCES

Alzheimer's Association: 2018 Alzheimer's disease facts and figures. Alzheimers Dement 14(3):367–429 2018

Bragg EJ, Warshaw GA, Meganathan K, Brewer DE: National survey of geriatric medicine fellowship programs: comparing findings in 2006/07 and 2001/02 from the American Geriatrics Society and Association of Directors of Geriatric Academic Programs Geriatrics Workforce Policy Studies Center. J Am Geriatr Soc 58(11):2166–2172 2010 21039369

Bragg EJ, Wasrshaw GA, Cheong J et al: National survey of geriatric psychiatry fellowship programs: comparing findings in 2006/07 and 2001/02 from the American Geriatrics Society and Association of Directors of Geriatric Academic Programs' Geriatrics Workforce Policy Studies Center. Am J Geriatr Psychiatry 20(2):169–178 2012 22273737

Institute of Medicine: Retooling for an Aging America: Building the Health Care Workforce. Washington, DC, National Academies Press, 2008

Institute of Medicine: The Mental Health and Substance Use Workforce for Older Adults: In Whose Hands? Washington, DC, The National Academies Press, 2012

PREFACE

A person with dementia not only loses memories and the ability to care for herself. She may become depressed or anxious, understandably apprehensive about her illness. Her bewildered family members may wonder why she is accusing them of stealing from her or why she says she sees her dead parents in her room at night. The staff of the assisted living facility where she lives may call her doctor's office for urgent help because she has just struck another resident.

Alzheimer's disease and other causes of dementia are classified as neuro*cognitive* disorders—but they are also very much disorders of *emotion* and *behavior*. Over 90% of people with dementia experience behavioral and psychological symptoms at some point during their illness (Kales et al. 2014). These symptoms profoundly affect quality of life, relationships with loved ones, personal safety, autonomy, dignity, and independence. Behavioral and psychological symptoms sometimes arise unpredictably, with terrible timing, when a family is already struggling to address the cognitive and functional consequences of dementia. Unfortunately, managing these symptoms is difficult, with few interventions that are effective and safe.

The purpose of this book is to provide readers with evidence-based, pragmatic, and clear recommendations regarding the care of patients with behavioral and psychological symptoms of dementia (BPSD). The book begins with an overview of dementia and its assessment and then moves on to a framework for the overall management of dementia. The core of the book details the assessment and management of BPSD; in other words, it tries to answer the question, "What should I do when my patient with dementia has a behavior that is affecting her quality of life or safety?" The book closes with addressing other threats to safety (e.g., falls, wandering), and ethical and legal considerations. Each chapter opens with a paragraph-long précis to orient the reader. Each chapter concludes with key points that encapsulate what to take away from the chapter and a list of resources that the reader can share with patients, families, and caregivers and references to the evidence base for the recommendations made.

This book is intended for any clinician who cares for people with dementia. In researching and writing this book, I drew on the (sometimes not too satisfying) literature on BPSD and on my 15 years of experience working with patients with dementia and their families and teaching others who do the same. I have taught primary care providers, psychiatrists, neurologists, and residents in psychiatry, neurology, family medicine, internal medicine, and emergency medicine, so these are the readers I envisioned as I wrote the book. I hope that others involved in the care of older adults with dementia and their families—for example, nurses, social workers, and psychologists—will also find the book useful. I hope above all that the burden of having dementia or caring for someone with dementia can be lifted, at least a little bit.

Art Walaszek, M.D.
Madison, Wisconsin
August 2018

REFERENCE

Kales HC, Gitlin LN, Lyketsos CG: Management of neuropsychiatric symptoms of dementia in clinical settings: recommendations from a multidisciplinary expert panel. J Am Geriatr Soc 62(4):762–769, 2014 24635665

ACKNOWLEDGMENTS

I am first and foremost indebted to the many mentors who instilled in me a passion for caring for older adults with dementia and their family members. An admittedly incomplete list includes Cheryl Woodson, Mark Snowden, Marcella Pascualy, Tim Howell, and Sanjay Asthana.

I have been very fortunate to have roles in the Wisconsin Alzheimer's Disease Research Center and the Wisconsin Alzheimer's Institute, both of which have supported my efforts to teach others about behavioral and psychological symptoms of dementia. These roles have brought me many friends and colleagues and much joy.

Although this book appears to be a work by a single author, it was, in fact, informed and shaped by the many discussions I have had with colleagues over the years about how best to care for patients with behavioral and psychological symptoms of dementia. I am especially obliged to Mark Snowden, Lisa Boyle, Eileen Ahearn, Ike Ahmed, and Lucy Wang, who thoughtfully reviewed the manuscript as it took shape.

I am grateful for the patience and trust of my colleagues at American Psychiatric Association Publishing—namely, Laura Roberts and John McDuffie.

Of course, I would be nowhere and nobody without the unconditional support of my family: Maddy, Lucy, Dewey, Percy, and—obviously—Suzanne.

CHAPTER 1

OVERVIEW OF DEMENTIA

Précis

The first step in understanding and addressing behavioral and psychological symptoms of dementia (BPSD) is establishing the cause of dementia. The nature of the symptoms varies based on the cause of dementia; the cause also influences the selection of treatment. For example, patients with dementia with Lewy bodies (DLB) may experience very vivid visual hallucinations, and they can be prone to developing side effects from antipsychotics. The most common cause of dementia is Alzheimer's disease (AD), and most of the research on treating BPSD has been conducted with subjects with AD. Other common dementias include Lewy body disease (DLB and Parkinson disease dementia [PDD]), vascular dementia, and frontotemporal dementia (FTD). The diagnostic evaluation includes identifying comorbid conditions contributing to cognitive impairment, such as depression, hypothyroidism, vitamin deficiency, electrolyte imbalance, alcohol use, and medication side effects. Ideally, the diagnosis will have been determined prior to the onset of BPSD; realistically, the clinician addressing acute BPSD may need to start with a focused diagnostic evaluation, initiate treatment of acute BPSD, and then conduct a more thorough diagnostic evaluation once the patient's distress has improved and safety has been ensured.

BACKGROUND AND TERMINOLOGY

Dementia is a progressive condition that affects cognition and functioning. Most patients with dementia also experience changes in emotion, personality, and behavior. In DSM-5 (American Psychiatric Association 2013), the term *major neurocognitive disorder* is preferred to *dementia*. Both terms are acceptable, and *dementia* is used most often in this book. In DSM-5, the etiology is then specified as in, for example, "major neurocognitive disorder due to Alzheimer's disease," and then further specified as "with behavioral disturbance" or "without behavioral disturbance."

The *major* in major neurocognitive disorder indicates that the cognitive deficits produce functional impairment and distinguishes it from *mild neurocognitive disorder*, which consists of cognitive decline but not significant functional decline. Patients with mild neurocognitive disorder may experience only slight impairments in activities of daily livings (ADLs), or they may be able to complete all ADLs but have a harder time doing so. Synonyms for mild neurocognitive disorder include *mild cognitive impairment* (MCI) and *cognitive impairment no dementia* (CIND). MCI is used throughout this book. It is probably simplest to think of MCI as the stage prior to dementia; for example, persons with AD progress from cognitive intactness (in which biological markers of AD may be present but there is no evidence of cognitive impairment) to MCI (in which cognition, but not functioning, is beginning to be impaired) to dementia (in which cognition is more impaired and functioning is also impaired). See Figure 1–1 for a graphical representation.

Although the following information is a bit beyond the scope of this book, it is worth noting that there are several subtypes of MCI, which may help with determining the underlying etiology (Petersen et al. 2009). The primary deficit in *amnestic MCI* (aMCI) is memory; people with aMCI are much more likely to "convert" to dementia due to AD than are people with other types of MCI or without MCI. Therefore, aMCI is thought to be an early manifestation of AD, prior to the onset of dementia. *Multiple domain MCI* (mdMCI) may or may not include memory loss, has a much less clear prognosis than aMCI (specifically, some people with mdMCI never progress, and others revert to normal cognition), and has a broader differential diagnosis than aMCI (e.g., cerebrovascular disease, depression).

This would be a good time to explore what exactly is meant by *cognition*. Cognition consists of several domains or functions, each of which has associated dysfunctions:

- *Memory:* The encoding (storing) and retrieving (recalling) of memories, which may be verbal, visual, or procedural (e.g., tying one's shoes). A deficit of memory is called *amnesia. Anterograde amnesia* is a problem with encoding new memories; *retrograde amnesia* is a problem with recalling old memories.
- *Attention:* The ability to maintain focus on a stimulus or task and shifting to a more relevant stimulus when warranted.

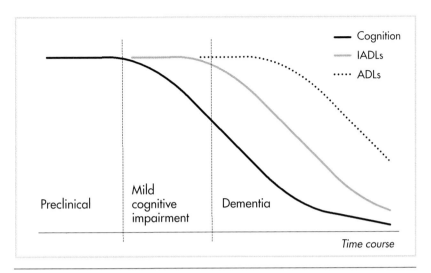

FIGURE 1–1. Course of dementia.

During the *preclinical* phase, cognition is intact and the ability to perform instrumental activities of daily living (IADLs) and activities of daily living (ADLs) is intact; biomarkers of the underlying etiology may be present (see Figure 1–3). In *mild cognitive impairment* (or mild neurocognitive disorder), cognitive abilities begin to decline; although functioning remains intact, more effort may be required to perform IADLs. In *dementia* (or major neurocognitive disorder), both cognition and functioning are impaired; the ability to perform IADLs declines first, followed by the ability to perform ADLs.

- *Language:* The understanding and production of speech and written language. A person with a *receptive* (fluent) *aphasia* has a problem with understanding language, whereas a person with an *expressive* (nonfluent) *aphasia* has difficulty speaking and writing; some people will have both.
- *Visuospatial function:* The processing of visual information, including what an object is and where it is in space. *Hemispatial neglect*, wherein one is unable to attend to visual stimuli on one side, is an example of dysfunction of the visuospatial system. Another example is *agnosia*, which refers to difficulty recognizing objects or faces.
- *Praxis:* The ability to perform complex motor tasks (e.g., buttoning a shirt). *Apraxia* refers to difficulty with complex motor tasks despite otherwise intact sensory and motor systems.
- *Executive function:* The ability to process and act on incoming information. This includes sequencing (e.g., putting on pants before shoes), planning and strategizing, initiating actions, impulse control, judgment, and cognitive flexibility (being able to change plans as circumstances change).

- *Social cognition:* The ability to interact with and understand other people. Abnormalities in interpersonal functioning may include lack of concern about or for others, lack of inhibitions in interactions with others, and inability to appreciate the mental states of others.

Another common cognitive abnormality in dementia is *anosognosia*, or lack of awareness that one has a problem; in a mental health context, this might be called *lack of insight*.

The hallmark of major neurocognitive disorder that distinguishes it from mild neurocognitive disorder is impairment in ADLs. There are two categories of ADLs: instrumental and personal (or basic) (Katz 1983). The instrumental ADLs (IADLs) are higher-order functions that tend to be affected earlier in the course of dementia. The mnemonic SHAFT covers the IADLs (University of Ottawa 2014):

S = Shopping for groceries, clothes, and other household items
H = Housekeeping
A = Accounting—that is, managing one's finances, including paying bills
F = Food preparation
T = Transportation—not necessarily driving, but more broadly the ability to get around, whether by cab or bus or by driving oneself

A person who cannot complete his or her basic or personal ADLs might die without assistance. The mnemonic DEATH is useful for remembering the personal ADLs (University of Ottawa 2014):

D = Dressing oneself
E = Eating—that is, feeding oneself
A = Ambulating
T = Toileting
H = Hygiene

People with dementia may also have a hard time managing their medications, which can hamper the effectiveness of interventions and can result in safety problems. Examples of medication management problems include taking too much medication (perhaps because a patient forgets having already taken it), taking too little medication (forgetting to take it), or taking medication irregularly. (This topic is covered more extensively in Chapter 6.)

Note that a patient with dementia may also have other ailments that affect functioning and compound the impairments associated with dementia. For example, vision impairment (quite common in older adults, who are prone to glaucoma, cataracts, macular degeneration, and diabetic retinopathy), osteoarthritis (which about half of older adults have), peripheral neuropathy, parkinsonism, depression, anxiety, and alcohol use can also profoundly affect the ability to complete ADLs.

CAUSES OF DEMENTIA

Significant cognitive and functional decline is never due simply to aging. Most commonly, patients with dementia have a neurodegenerative disorder such as AD, Lewy body disease, or FTD. Cerebrovascular disease is another common etiology, often comorbid with a neurodegenerative process. Head injury, normal pressure hydrocephalus, alcohol, anticholinergic medications, electrolyte imbalance, depression, and anxiety also may contribute to cognitive impairment. The major etiologies are compared in Table 1–1.

Establishing the cause of dementia is not simply an academic exercise. In some cases, a reversible etiology may be found—and when this etiology is addressed, the patient's cognition and functioning can improve. The diagnosis influences the presentation of symptoms; for example, patients with Lewy body disease may experience very vivid visual hallucinations, whereas patients with FTD may be disinhibited and physically aggressive. Perhaps most importantly, the treatment plan may vary based on diagnosis. Although it may be tempting to prescribe antipsychotics to try to address hallucinations in a patient with Lewy body disease, this in fact could result in the patient's condition worsening.

The clinician interested in a more in-depth discussion of the causes of dementia should continue reading; other readers should feel free to skip to the next section, "Assessment of Dementia."

Alzheimer's Disease

AD (in DSM-5 parlance, major neurocognitive disorder due to AD) is a neurodegenerative disorder that affects memory, language, visuospatial function, and executive function and that ultimately results in progressive decline in ability to conduct ADLs. The pathological hallmarks of AD are *amyloid plaques* and *neurofibrillary tangles* accompanied by inflammation (Sperling et al. 2011). Amyloid plaques consist of "bad" β-amyloid and form outside of neurons, disrupting neuronal connections. Amyloid precursor protein (APP) is a normal constituent of neuronal cell membranes and normally gets cleaved into nonpathological, soluble β-amyloid. The amyloid hypothesis—namely, that the abnormal cleaving of APP into "bad" β-amyloid

TABLE 1–1. Comparison of the major causes of dementia

Cause of dementia	Course and cognitive symptoms	Behavioral and psychological symptoms
Alzheimer's disease	Slow, progressive decline, typically in this order: memory, language, visuospatial function, executive function	Mild dementia: depression, anxiety, insomnia Moderate to severe dementia: hallucinations, delusions, repetitiveness, aggression
Lewy body disease: dementia with Lewy bodies (DLB), Parkinson disease dementia (PDD)	Slow, progressive decline but with fluctuations in cognition reminiscent of delirium; memory deficit; visuospatial dysfunction; motor symptoms precede cognitive impairment in PDD, less significant in DLB; sensitivity to side effects of antipsychotics	Visual hallucinations, delusions, anxiety, rapid eye movement sleep behavior disorder
Vascular dementia	Classically, a stepwise progression (but not always detectable clinically); affected cognitive domains depend on location of vascular lesions	Apathy, amotivation, depression
Frontotemporal dementia, behavioral variant	Relatively rapid decline, affects younger patients (45–64 years old); significant language deficits and executive dysfunction	Disinhibition, verbal repetitiveness, verbal aggression, physical aggression, hyperorality, apathy

is the first step in the pathophysiological cascade of AD—is currently the most widely accepted hypothesis explaining how AD arises (Figure 1–2).

Neurofibrillary tangles are located within neurons and consist of hyperphosphorylated tau protein. Normally, tau protein is associated with microtubules and makes up the skeletal structure of a neuron; when tau gets hyperphosphorylated, it tangles and clumps into neurofibrillary tangles, a process that then results in the death of neurons (Dubois et al. 2007). (For

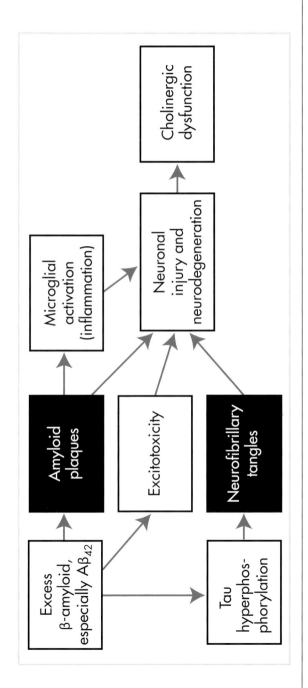

FIGURE 1–2. How Alzheimer's disease (AD) arises.

According to the amyloid hypothesis, excess accumulation of β-amyloid is the first step in the development of AD. Aβ$_{42}$ ("bad" amyloid) aggregates into extracellular amyloid plaques, one of the two neuropathological hallmarks of AD. Plaques are accompanied by an inflammatory response mediated by microglial activation. β-Amyloid may result in hyperphosphorylation of the protein tau (although how this happens is unclear), which in turn aggregates into intracellular neurofibrillary tangles, the other neuropathological hallmark of AD. β-Amyloid is also excitotoxic. All of these factors (plaques, tangles, inflammation, excitotoxicity) lead to neuronal injury and death. A final downstream step is a deficit of cholinergic transmission due to death of cholinergic neurons.

this reason, AD is sometimes referred to as a tauopathy.) It is not clear how the abnormal amyloid and tau processes are related to each other: does one cause the other, or are both the consequences of another process?

Inflammation accompanies the formation of plaques and therefore is essentially a maladaptive response to what are, in effect, foreign bodies (McGeer and McGeer 2001). Microglia, the macrophages of the central nervous system, are responsible for inflammatory responses within the brain: when activated, microglia clear amyloid deposits but also release cytotoxic inflammatory factors, which results in cell death and increases the amount of β-amyloid.

The hippocampus and medial temporal lobes, areas involved in encoding memories, are the first to be affected, specifically by neurofibrillary tangles (Dubois et al. 2007). Therefore, memory deficits arise first. The pathology then spreads to the remainder of the temporal lobes and to the parietal lobes, affecting language and visuospatial function, respectively. Finally, the frontal lobes are affected, resulting in executive dysfunction. Structural neuroimaging (magnetic resonance imaging [MRI] and computed tomography [CT]) can detect this sequence of events, by showing atrophy of gray and white matter and increased cerebrospinal fluid signal (*ex vacuo* changes) (Ahmed et al. 2014). Functional neuroimaging (fluorodeoxyglucose positron emission tomography [FDG-PET]) can detect these changes even earlier by identifying areas of the brain with decreased metabolism. New imaging techniques that would allow for detection of amyloid and tau proteins are being studied (Ahmed et al. 2014).

The pathological changes associated with AD may begin 20 or more years before symptoms first appear. Therefore, the term *Alzheimer's disease* currently encompasses a continuum that includes patients with no clinical findings whatsoever, patients with MCI (cognitive impairment but no functional impairment), and patients with dementia (the end stage of AD). This raises the possibility that medical professionals will be able to identify patients at risk of developing dementia and intervene to reduce this risk.

In fact, a critical area of research in AD is discovering biomarkers to identify people during the preclinical stage of the disease. As best as researchers can tell, markers of abnormal amyloid metabolism appear first, then markers of tau hyperphosphorylation emerge, then comes neuronal injury and neurodegeneration (Sperling et al. 2011) (Figure 1–3). The A/T/N classification system of biomarkers captures this and allows for the description of dementias not due to AD (Jack et al. 2016):

- "A" refers to amyloid biomarkers: the identification of excess amyloid on amyloid PET imaging; low levels of Aβ$_{42}$ in cerebrospinal fluid. Abnor-

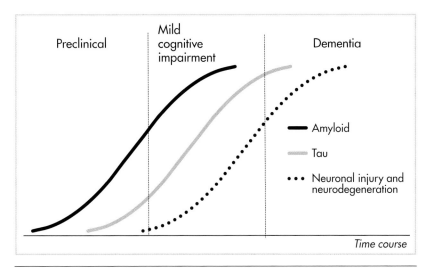

FIGURE 1–3. Biomarkers in Alzheimer's disease.

In Alzheimer's disease, markers of abnormal amyloid metabolism are thought to arise first, followed by markers of tau hyperphosphorylation, and then by markers of neuronal injury and neurodegeneration (e.g., abnormal neuroimaging). See text for details. Note that the divisions between the preclinical phase, mild cognitive impairment, and dementia with respect to biomarkers are approximate, because these states are currently defined clinically (see Figure 1.1) rather than by pathophysiology or pathology.

Source. Adapted from Sperling et al. 2011.

malities in amyloid metabolism may be the earliest findings in AD but are also not necessarily specific to AD.

- "T" refers to tau biomarkers: the identification of tau on tau PET imaging; high levels of phosphorylated tau in cerebrospinal fluid. Phosphorylated tau is quite specific to AD and rarely seen in other causes of dementia.
- "N" refers to neuronal injury and neurodegeneration: high levels of total tau in cerebrospinal fluid (a general marker of neuronal injury, seen in many causes of dementia); hypometabolism demonstrated on FDG-PET; atrophy demonstrated on CT or MRI. In AD, the temporal and parietal lobes are usually affected, whereas other regions are affected in other causes of dementia.

For example, A+/T+/N– means that an asymptomatic person has preclinical AD, with amyloid and tau biomarkers present, but no evidence of neuronal injury or neurodegeneration yet; this person would be at risk of developing MCI and then dementia. Interestingly, many people with Alzheimer's pathology (or other pathology, as described in later sections) never go on to develop dementia clinically. Conversely, some people with clinical diagnoses of dementia due to AD turn out to not have extensive Alzheimer's pathology and do not appear to benefit from treatments targeting Alzheimer's pathology. Clearly, more work needs to be to done to correlate pathology and the clinical symptoms of dementia.

As of 2017, about 5.5 million Americans had AD; this number is projected to nearly triple by 2050 (Alzheimer's Association 2017). Most people with AD are ages 75–84 years, although the number over age 85 is growing rapidly. More women than men have AD, with a proportion of about 1.7:1. African Americans and Hispanics are more likely to develop AD than non-Hispanic whites, and there is emerging evidence that the risk of AD is fairly high among American Indians (Mayeda et al. 2016).

The most powerful risk factors for AD are age and family history (Alzheimer's Association 2017). Among those ages 65–74 years, the prevalence of AD is 3%; among those ages 75–84 years, it is 17%; and among those age 85 years and older, it is 32%. Having one or more parents or siblings with AD increases the risk of developing AD. Other risk factors include fewer years of formal education, traumatic brain injury, depression, cardiovascular risk factors (e.g., smoking, diabetes, obesity, hypertension, high cholesterol), physical inactivity during midlife, and hearing loss.

The most common genetic risk factor for AD is the ε4 allele of the apolipoprotein E (*APOE*) mutation (Alzheimer's Association 2017; Sperling et al. 2011). About one-quarter of the U.S. population carries either one or two copies of the ε4 allele. Carrying one copy of this allele increases the risk of developing AD threefold (relative to not carrying any copies), and carrying two copies results in 8–12 times increased risk. Another way of conceptualizing this risk is the following: an ε4 carrier would be expected to develop AD 5–10 years earlier than a noncarrier. It should be noted that *APOE* does not fully account for the risk associated with family history—thus far, more than 20 genetic risk factors have been identified (Ahmed et al. 2014).

The most powerful, but thankfully rare, genetic risk factors for AD are mutations of the APP gene (which encodes amyloid precursor protein) and the Presenilin-1 and Presenilin-2 genes (*PS1* and *PS2*, which encode enzymes involved in the cleavage of amyloid precursor protein) (Ahmed et al. 2014). All carriers of these autosomal dominant and highly penetrant mutations will develop early-onset AD. Finally, about 30% of people with Down syndrome who are in their 50s have AD: the APP gene is on chromosome 21, of which people with Down syndrome have three copies, leading to overproduction of amyloid.

Clinicians should be aware of two conditions related to AD: *posterior cortical atrophy* and *cerebral amyloid angiopathy*. Patients with posterior cortical atrophy have neurodegeneration in their parietal, occipital, and temporal cortices, resulting in problems with reading, navigating, and identifying objects due to cortical blindness; they are typically younger than patients with AD, and memory problems develop later than in AD (Suárez-González et al. 2015). Cerebral amyloid angiopathy is characterized by the deposition of amyloid in blood vessels within the brain, resulting in hemorrhagic infarcts and a course more akin to vascular dementia (see later subsection) than AD (Charidimou et al. 2012).

Treating AD requires a comprehensive plan to enhance cognition, educate and support patients and their families, support ADLs, address safety issues, prevent elder abuse, and plan for the future—all topics covered in Chapter 2. A comprehensive plan will also address behavioral and psychological symptoms—the topic of the remainder of this book.

Lewy Body Disease

Lewy bodies are abnormal deposits of the protein α-synuclein within neurons and are characteristic of the two major types of Lewy body disease: PDD and DLB (McKeith et al. 2017). (Along with multiple system atrophy, these conditions are collectively referred to as synucleinopathies because of their common neuropathology.) Patients with Parkinson disease first develop the classic motor symptoms of rigidity, bradykinesia, tremor, and postural instability. As the disease progresses, cognitive impairment eventually develops, including memory loss, slowed processing speed, and inattention.

In patients with DLB, cognitive symptoms are more prominent early and may include cognitive fluctuation severe enough to mimic delirium; Lewy bodies are found within the cerebral cortex as opposed to subcortical regions (McKeith et al. 2017). Psychiatric symptoms such as vivid visual hallucinations are common. Tremor tends to be less severe than in PDD. Patients may develop rapid eye movement (REM) sleep behavior disorder, characterized by nighttime vocalizations and behavioral disturbance, prior to the onset of other symptoms (McKeith et al. 2017). Patients with DLB demonstrate exquisite sensitivity to antipsychotics, becoming markedly parkinsonian when exposed to antipsychotics; other possible symptoms include postural instability, repeated falls, syncope, autonomic dysfunction, hypersomnia, nonvisual hallucinations, delusions, apathy, anxiety, and depression (collectively referred to as "supportive clinical features" in the diagnosis of DLB).

Biomarkers do not yet have widespread clinical use in diagnosing Lewy body disease. They include reduced dopamine transporter uptake in the basal ganglia, as demonstrated by single-photon emission computed tomography (SPECT) or PET (sensitivity and specificity of 80% and 90%, respectively, in distinguishing from AD); abnormal [123]iodine-metaiodobenzylguanidine (MIBG) myocardial scintigraphy, which is due to reduced sympathetic innervation of the heart (sensitivity and specificity of 69% and 87% when distinguishing from AD); and polysomnography indicating REM sleep without atonia, which is very specific for Lewy body disease (Ahmed et al. 2014; McKeith et al. 2017). Nonspecific but potentially useful biomarkers include relative preservation of medial temporal lobes on structural neuroimaging (atrophy would suggest AD instead); hypometabolism in the occipital lobes on FDG-PET; and an abnormal electroencephalogram.

Distinguishing between Lewy body disease and other causes of dementia is important because treatment may include antiparkinsonian agents and should include cholinesterase inhibitors. In addition, because of the prominent psychotic symptoms of DLB, many patients with DLB come to psychiatric attention and are prescribed antipsychotics, which may exacerbate DLB, as illustrated in Case Example 1–1. See Chapter 5 for more on the problems associated with using antipsychotics in patients with DLB.

Case Example 1–1: "Big, Fuzzy Spiders"

Mrs. Sanchez, an 82-year old woman living alone in an apartment, was brought by her children to her primary care provider because of what appeared to be unfounded concern about an insect infestation. About 1 year earlier, she had begun complaining to her landlord and to her family that she saw insects in her bed. Insect exterminators had been sent to her apartment twice but found no evidence of an infestation. She started calling her children in the middle of the night because she would wake up, go to the bathroom, and see "big, fuzzy spiders" in the sink and toilet. After believing that there were insects in her food, Mrs. Sanchez began to eat less—she would eat only prepackaged foods—and lost 15 pounds in 6 months. Her children also noticed that she was not taking good care of herself or the apartment, which they thought was due to her preoccupation with insects. She had also fallen twice, though without injury. Her medical history included dyslipidemia (for which she was taking lovastatin), osteoarthritis (ibuprofen, as needed), hiatal hernia (omeprazole), chronic constipation (various stool softeners), and insomnia (over-the-counter hypnotic). The physical examination was notable for unsteady gait but was otherwise reported to be normal.

The primary care provider ordered the following tests: basic metabolic panel, complete blood count, thyroid-stimulating hormone, and rapid plasma reagin. All were negative. A CT scan of the head showed global atrophy, somewhat more than expected for her age. Suspecting that the insects represented visual hallucinations due to psychosis and that Mrs. Sanchez had developed schizophrenia, the physician recommended risperidone, 1 mg at bedtime, and placed a referral to a psychiatrist for further management.

During the wait for the psychiatric evaluation, Mrs. Sanchez's condition worsened. She was now falling once a week, and her family was advised to find an assisted living facility for her. Her family wondered if she had become depressed, because they noticed that she was moving more slowly and her facial expression seemed blank. The hallucinations did not improve—in fact, she was now becoming suspicious of others and had to be coaxed into allowing her children to come into her apartment. The primary care provider increased risperidone to 2 mg at bedtime.

Mrs. Sanchez's children were distraught by the time of the psychiatric evaluation, alarmed at her deterioration over the past 18 months. The psychiatrist noted that Mrs. Sanchez was guarded in her responses to questions and somewhat preoccupied. She was disoriented to time, was amnestic for recent events, and scored 15 out of 30 on the Saint Louis University Mental Status (SLUMS; Tariq et al. 2006) examination. She had masked facies and a resting tremor affecting the right arm more than the left arm. She had cogwheeling in both arms, had difficulty getting out of her chair, and walked with a shuffling gait. Suspecting that Mrs. Sanchez's parkinsonism was due to risperidone, the psychiatrist recommended discontinuing it; she also recommended discontinuing the hypnotic agent, believing that this was contributing to hallucinations and memory loss.

At the next appointment 1 month later, Mrs. Sanchez's parkinsonism had improved but not resolved—she still had a resting tremor and cogwheeling in her right arm, and her gait was still shuffling. Her memory had improved slightly, and her SLUMS score was now 18 out of 30. She was no longer taking risperidone or the hypnotic. But Mrs. Sanchez was still seeing insects throughout her apartment, and she remained paranoid. It now appeared that DLB was the likely cause of Mrs. Sanchez's cognitive and functional decline and visual hallucinations. The psychiatrist recommended a trial of donepezil 5 mg/day, titrated to 10 mg/day after 1 month.

Two months later, the patient's visual hallucinations had nearly completely resolved (she still saw what looked like insects in her peripheral vision once in a while at night), and she was no longer paranoid. She had fallen only once in the past 2 months. Her memory had continued to improve, and her SLUMS score was now 20 out of 30. Mrs. Sanchez was now doing better with respect to personal ADLs. However, because Mrs. Sanchez remained behind on her bills, was unable to resume cooking on her own, and was up quite a bit at night, the psychiatrist advised that she get increased support at home.

Vascular Dementia

Cerebrovascular risk factors—hypertension, dyslipidemia, diabetes mellitus, and obesity—contribute to the risk of both AD and vascular dementia (referred to as major vascular neurocognitive disorder in DSM-5, and formerly called multi-infarct dementia) (O'Brien and Thomas 2015). In fact, as discussed later, AD and vascular dementia commonly coexist. The classic story of vascular dementia is that of a patient who has a stepwise decline in cognition and functioning, with each step resulting from a stroke. The reality is more complex, because patients with vascular dementia seem to fall into three camps: 1) those with discrete "steps"; 2) those who have a devastating stroke (e.g., infarction in the territory of the left middle cerebral artery, which may result in expressive aphasia and a dense right hemiplegia) and do indeed experience a "step," albeit a very large one; and 3) those with many small infarcts (often seen as white matter changes in periventricular regions and in the white matter tracts leading to and from the frontal lobes or as lacunes within deeper structures), each of which is not widespread enough to cause a noticeable "step" but which collectively result in cognitive and functional decline. Other conditions that fall into the constellation of vascular dementia include cerebral amyloid angiopathy (discussed earlier in the subsection on Alzheimer's disease) and CADASIL (cerebral autosomal dominant arteriopathy with subcortical infarcts and leukoencephalopathy), which causes severe ischemic disease due to a mutation in the notch3 gene (O'Brien and Thomas 2015). In other words, the term *vascular dementia* refers to a wide range of somewhat disparate conditions. The term *vascular cognitive impairment* is sometimes used to refer to a continuum of presentations, from MCI to dementia, due to cerebrovascular disease (O'Brien and Thomas 2015). Patients with MCI who experience decline in multiple cognitive domains (one of which may be memory) may go on to develop vascular dementia (Petersen et al. 2009).

The exact nature of the cognitive symptoms in vascular dementia depends on the location of the infarct(s). Anterograde amnesia (inability to form new memories) alone is less common in vascular dementia than in AD, because the hippocampus and medial temporal lobes are unlikely to experience ischemia in the absence of other regions being affected. However, retrieval of memory, largely a frontal lobe function, may become problematic in patients with vascular dementia. Aphasia and executive dysfunction are fairly common, as is apathy, which may mimic depression; note the related construct of "vascular depression," which usually refers to the late-life onset of depressive symptoms, characterized by apathy, anergia, and anhedonia but not necessarily dysphoria, guilt, or worthlessness. The neurological examination of a patient with vascular dementia will be abnormal, and neuroimaging findings (CT or MRI) should correlate with physical examination findings.

Mixed Dementia

Many patients with AD also have cerebrovascular disease or Lewy bodies or both. Most patients with Lewy body disease and vascular dementia also have Alzheimer's pathology. Collectively, this is referred to as "mixed dementia" (McKhann et al. 2011; O'Brien and Thomas 2015). Mixed dementia is quite common. Although the literature is somewhat contradictory, it appears that patients with both AD and DLB do worse than those with AD alone, whereas those with both AD and vascular dementia have a less severe course than with AD alone. The point for the busy clinician is that mixed dementia is nearly as common as "pure" forms of dementia, a fact that complicates diagnosis and treatment.

Frontotemporal Dementia

FTD is characterized by changes in behavior or speech due to focal degeneration of the frontal or temporal lobes (Bang et al. 2015). It is a particularly devastating cause of dementia because it afflicts relatively young people— 60% of patients with FTD have onset between ages 45 and 64 years—with profound effects on ability to work and on family life. Onset is insidious, as in other neurodegenerative causes of dementia, but the course tends to be rapid—about 2–5 years from diagnosis to death.

Clinically, there are two major presentations of FTD, the behavioral variant and the language variant (Bang et al. 2015). The behavioral variant includes Pick's disease, first described in the late nineteenth century and characterized pathologically by Pick bodies (discussed later in this section). The classic symptoms of the behavioral variant include disinhibition (manifest as socially inappropriate behavior, inappropriate sexual comments, verbal aggression, physical aggression, impulsive decision making), apathy, hyperorality (e.g., eating excessively, craving sweets or carbohydrates, rigid preferences for specific foods, trying to eat things that are not food), and repetitive speech or behaviors (sometimes misconstrued as the compulsions of obsessive-compulsive behavior). Many of these symptoms reflect disturbances of social cognition, as described earlier (see the section "Background and Terminology"). The language variant, also called *primary progressive aphasia* (PPA), is notable for prominent word-finding difficulties, impaired naming, and impaired language comprehension (Bang et al. 2015). *Semantic dementia* is also a language variant of FTD and is notable for patients losing the meaning associated with words (Bang et al. 2015). As PPA and semantic dementia progress, executive dysfunction and eventually global cognitive impairment occur, and behavioral symptoms can emerge.

Related clinical entities for clinicians to be aware of include *progressive supranuclear palsy* (PSP), *corticobasal degeneration* (CBD), and *FTD with motor neuron disease* (Dickson 2009). The symptoms of PSP include apathy, disinhibition, vertical gaze ophthalmoplegia, axial rigidity, and frequent falls. CBD symptoms include akinesia, rigidity, propensity to fall, apraxia, dystonia, and alien limb syndrome. Patients with PSP and CBD can appear similar to those with Parkinson disease, such that PSP and CBD used to be thought of as "Parkinson-plus" syndromes; in fact, however, PSP and CBD are pathologically more closely related to FTD. Levodopa tends not be effective in addressing the parkinsonism found in PSP and CBD. Finally, it used to be thought that patients with motor neuron disease such as amyotrophic lateral sclerosis were spared cognitive impairment; in fact, upper and lower motor neuron signs are not uncommon in FTD, especially the behavioral variant.

The neuropathology of FTD is complex (Dickson 2009). Most cases of FTD are due to either abnormalities of the tau protein (the protein implicated in AD) or a protein called TDP-43 (TAR DNA-binding protein with a molecular weight of 43 kilodaltons). Pick bodies, neuronal inclusion bodies rich with tau protein, are commonly found in the behavioral variant of FTD; tau is also involved in the pathophysiology of PSP and most cases of CBD; hence, like AD, these are tauopathies. Abnormalities of TDP-43 are found in most cases of the language variant of FTD, most cases of FTD with motor neuron disease, some cases of CBD, and some cases of the behavioral variant of FTD. The exact details of the genetic contributions to FTD are beyond the scope of this book but suffice it to say that 40% of patients with FTD have a family history of dementia, and 10% of patients with FTD appear to have an autosomal dominant mutation (Bang et al. 2015).

Why is any of this information relevant in a book on the BPSD? The various forms of FTD (including PPA, as it progresses) pose significant challenges because patients, families, and other caregivers must contend with sometimes severe behavioral problems (aggression, disinhibition, impulsivity, hypersexual behavior) in fairly young and sometimes otherwise healthy adults and the attendant risks to the safety of the patient and others. The data on effective treatment of behavioral symptoms in FTD are more sparse than the data on treatment of such symptoms in AD, making FTD a particularly challenging condition for clinicians to treat. With its midlife onset and prominent behavioral and psychological symptoms, FTD can mimic other psychiatric disorders such as major depressive disorder and bipolar disorder, as depicted in Case Example 1–2. So, it is important to keep FTD in the differential diagnosis of adults in their 50s and beyond presenting with depression or mania.

Case Example 1–2: "He's Embarrassing My Daughters and Me."

Mr. Erickson was a well-regarded high school principal until age 62, when he became increasingly withdrawn from his work and started to have problems completing all of his paperwork. His family thought that he was depressed, perhaps due to financial problems in the school district. Budget cuts had led to loss of his administrative staff, resulting in an increased workload for him. He was in good health, except for hypertension (well controlled with hydrochlorothiazide) and obesity (which had worsened recently—he had gained 20 pounds in 6 months). He had no prior psychiatric history. He drank one or two beers each night and did not use cannabis or any illicit substances. Following his family's advice, he saw a therapist for depression, and the therapist in turn referred him to a psychiatrist, who prescribed sertraline 50 mg/day. In a month, the dosage was increased to 100 mg/day. A thyroid-stimulating hormone test was normal.

After an initial improvement in mood, Mr. Erickson continued to have problems at work. He became yet more withdrawn after a teacher filed a complaint with the school board about insulting comments that Mr. Erickson had made to the teacher. Mr. Erickson received a poor performance review, and as a result he was notified that his job was in jeopardy. His family also noticed that he had started behaving erratically and impulsively, including blurting out comments about strangers and making several extravagant purchases. On one occasion, he made sexually inappropriate comments to his daughters' friends (something he had never done before), leading his wife to call the psychiatrist and complain, "He's embarrassing my daughters and me." The psychiatrist, concerned that sertraline had resulted in mania, discontinued sertraline and started quetiapine 50 mg/day, eventually titrated to 200 mg/day.

Owing to continued problems completing tasks at work, Mr. Erickson took a medical leave of absence. His family noted that he slept much of the day and did not participate in activities he used to enjoy, such as reading mystery novels and debating politics. He had become increasingly irritable and short-tempered; one day, his wife came home to find that he had smashed the television because he could not figure out how to turn it on. Six months after his initial assessment, he was not better—instead, he had continued to deteriorate. His family requested an evaluation at a memory clinic to determine the diagnosis.

Mr. Erickson's neurological examination was normal. His mental status examination was notable for word-finding difficulties, irritability, and mild disorientation to time. Mr. Erickson had abnormal bedside cognitive testing: he scored 20 out of 30 on the SLUMS examination, lower than expected for his educational attainment (master's degree) and occupation. His family was surprised to learn that he could not accurately draw a clock and that he could name only 11 animals in 1 minute. On the Patient Health Questionnaire–9 (PHQ-9; Spitzer et al. 1999), he scored 14, consistent with moderate depression. The neurologist ordered an MRI of the brain, which was read as normal for the patient's age. To distinguish between AD,

FTD, and depression, the neurologist ordered an FDG-PET scan, which revealed mild hypometabolism of bilateral frontal lobes and of the anterior pole of both temporal lobes—consistent with FTD.

The neurologist recommended that the patient be weaned from quetiapine, out of concern that sedation could be contributing to cognitive impairment. She also recommended that he stop drinking alcohol. The patient and his family were educated about the cause, course, and prognosis of FTD and referred to patient and caregiver support groups in the community.

Other Causes of Dementia

It should go without saying that excessive alcohol use has deleterious effects on brain health. Although there is some evidence that a low level of alcohol use (probably one standard drink per day or less) might be associated with a decreased risk of dementia, the net effect of alcohol on cognition is likely negative; once someone has developed dementia, further alcohol consumption worsens outcomes. The classic cognitive manifestations of heavy alcohol use include *Wernicke's encephalopathy* (an acute syndrome of confusion, ataxia, and ophthalmoplegia, reversible with administration of thiamine) and *Korsakoff's psychosis* (a chronic, typically irreversible condition characterized by profound anterograde amnesia and confabulation), which are collectively referred to as *Wernicke-Korsakoff syndrome* (Ridley et al. 2013). Thiamine deficiency resulting in degeneration of the mammillary bodies, thalamus, cerebellar hemispheres, and vermis is the cause of Wernicke-Korsakoff syndrome. The related syndrome of *alcohol-related dementia* appears to be due to a direct neurotoxic effect of alcohol, especially in the frontal lobes and basal forebrain (home of cholinergic neurons critical for attention and memory) and presents with impaired memory, visuospatial function, motor speed, and executive function, with relative sparing of language. (To further confuse matters, DSM-5 labels these entities as substance/medication-induced major or mild neurocognitive disorder; ICD-10 refers to them as alcohol-induced major or mild neurocognitive disorder, in which the major form has amnestic-confabulatory and nonamnestic-confabulatory types.) Whatever the label, abstinence can lead to improvements in cognition within a week and further recovery over the course of several years (Ridley et al. 2013).

The relationship between *traumatic brain injury* and acute cognitive impairment (i.e., concussion) has long been recognized (Alzheimer's Association 2017), but there is now increased awareness that repeated traumatic injury may result in persistent cognitive changes, with the most dramatic example being *chronic traumatic encephalopathy*, described primarily in participants of contact sports and in combat veterans. Behavioral and psychological symptoms, including suicidality, are prominent.

Patients with *normal pressure hydrocephalus* (NPH) present with cognitive impairment, falls, and urinary incontinence (a not uncommon combination in older adults, and so not particularly specific to NPH) (Shprecher et al. 2008). Neuroimaging reveals ventricles enlarged out of proportion to enlargement of sulci, and there is an elevated opening pressure during lumbar puncture; surgical shunting may help gait but tends not to improve cognition. The combination of falls and cognitive decline should also call to mind the possibility of *chronic subdural hematoma*: older adults are prone to subdural bleeding because brain atrophy results in the brain pulling away from the skull, leading to stretching of bridging veins, which in turn are susceptible to tearing when force is applied to the head, such as during a fall (Sahyouni et al. 2017). Symptoms of chronic subdural hematoma may manifest weeks after a head injury and may include cognitive impairment, headache, apathy, somnolence, and focal neurological deficits.

Creutzfeldt-Jakob disease (CJD) is a rare (annual incidence of about 1 in a million), rapidly progressive dementia, with death typically occurring within 1 year of diagnosis, caused by accumulation of prion protein (Glatzel et al. 2005). In addition to cognitive decline, patients with CJD often have myoclonus, insomnia (which can be quite severe), ataxia, nystagmus, and disturbance of mood. Cerebrospinal fluid levels of total tau protein are much higher in patients with CJD than in patients with AD and other conditions (Ahmed et al. 2014).

Neurosyphilis, once called the great imitator for its protean manifestations—depression, mania, psychosis, and dementia—is now uncommon, although it should be noted that rates of syphilis have been increasing since 2000 (Ghanem 2010). Untreated infection with *Treponema pallidum* can, 20–25 years later, result in amnesia, emotional lability, executive dysfunction, and confusion, in addition to the neurological symptoms of Argyll Robertson pupils and tabes dorsalis (demyelination of dorsal columns of the spinal cord, resulting in weakness, hyporeflexia, paresthesias, and loss of proprioception). Thankfully, HIV-associated dementia has also become quite uncommon, following the development of highly effective therapies for HIV (Clifford and Ances 2013). The classic symptoms included motor slowing, inattention, apathy, and depression; now, people living with HIV/AIDS are less likely to have severe cognitive and functional impairment, but they can show more subtle cognitive findings.

As discussed in the section "Assessment of Dementia," the diagnostic evaluation of a patient presenting with cognitive impairment includes a search for potentially reversible causes of dementia, especially delirium. It is important to consider these causes of cognitive impairment: medications (especially, anticholinergic medications, opioids, benzodiazepines, and other sedative-hypnotics), other substances (e.g., alcohol, cannabis), endocrine dysfunction (e.g., hypothyroidism or hyperthyroidism), metabolic disturbance (e.g., hyponatremia or hypernatremia, hypocalcemia or hypercalcemia, chronic kidney disease, liver disease [including hyperammonemia], hypoxia, hypercarbia, and hypoglycemia), vitamin deficiency (e.g., B_1, B_6, and especially B_{12}), and obstructive sleep apnea. Another critical mimic of dementia is depression; cognitive impairment due to depression in older adults is sometimes referred to as pseudodementia. It is possible that one of the reversible causes may still be superimposed on another cause (e.g., AD, cerebrovascular disease) and therefore that the cognitive and functional impairment may not be fully reversible. For example, hearing loss and visual impairment could contribute to cognitive impairment (by decreasing sensory inputs), but they are unlikely to be solely responsible. In fact, only around 1.5% of dementias have been found to be fully reversible (Harisingani 2005).

A Note on Pathology

Although not of immediate clinical relevance, an understanding of the neuropathology of dementia should be the key to discovering effective treatments for the various causes of dementia. For example, numerous potentially effective therapies for AD target amyloid protein. Figure 1–4 is a simplified schematic of the neuropathological causes of dementia and their associated clinical manifestations (Dickson 2009).

ASSESSMENT OF DEMENTIA

All older adults with cognitive and functional decline should undergo a diagnostic evaluation to identify the cause(s), including potentially reversible causes (Rabins et al. 2007). A patient presenting with BPSD may need to have a more limited evaluation at first, because the priority may be to rapidly stabilize the situation, but eventually, a more comprehensive evaluation should be completed. Patients and their families deserve a diagnosis and prognosis in order to promote their understanding of dementia and to help plan for the future (the latter topic is discussed further in Chapter 2). Please refer to Table 1–2 for an overview of assessment.

History and Examination

The diagnosis of dementia remains a clinical diagnosis, based on history from the patient and informants, physical examination, and mental status examination. The patient's capacity to understand and adhere to treatment

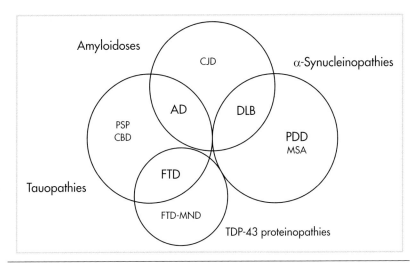

FIGURE 1–4. Neuropathology of dementia.

In addition to cerebrovascular disease and inflammation, the pathological hallmarks of dementia include disturbances in the proteins amyloid, tau, α-synuclein, and TDP-43 (TAR DNA-binding protein with a molecular weight of 43 kilodaltons), leading to amyloidoses, tauopathies, α-synucleinopathies, and TDP-43 proteinopathies, respectively. The relevant clinical entities include Alzheimer's disease (AD), corticobasal degeneration (CBD), Creutzfeldt-Jakob disease (CJD), dementia with Lewy bodies (DLB), frontotemporal dementia (FTD), frontotemporal dementia with motor neuron disease (FTD-MND), multisystem atrophy (MSA), Parkinson disease dementia (PDD), and progressive supranuclear palsy (PSP).

Source. Based on Dickson 2009.

of dementia may be a concern from the very first interaction. The assessment of decisional capacity and other capacities is discussed in Chapter 7.

History From the Patient

The clinician should elicit from the patient the nature, timing of onset, course, and severity of cognitive symptoms, including memory loss, word-finding difficulties, disorientation, inattention, and difficulty remembering others' names. Although dementia may limit the patient's ability to recall and discuss these symptoms, it is important that the clinician appreciate the patient's insight into his or her situation and learn what explanation the patient has for the symptoms. The patient should be asked about neurological symptoms that may aid in diagnosis, including gait difficulties or falls, focal weakness, vision loss, and hearing loss. A review of systems should also include, at the least, questioning about pain, gastrointestinal symptoms (changes in appetite, constipation, diarrhea), and urinary symptoms. As de-

TABLE 1–2.   Practical assessment of dementia

What?	How?	Why?
History from patient	Ask about nature, severity, and course of cognitive symptoms; screen for BPSD; conduct review of systems; assess ADLs; ask about use of alcohol and other substances; screen for elder abuse.	Develop hypothesis about possible etiologies, identify potential safety concerns, determine extent of functional impairment, assess risk of elder abuse.
History from caregiver(s)	Same as above; conduct together with patient or, if more appropriate or tolerable to patient, separately.	Corroborate and expand on patient's history.
Chart review	Review medical record, notes from patient's facility, notes from family or other caregivers, medication list, past medical and psychiatric history.	Refine hypothesis about possible etiologies, identify potential safety concerns, carefully assess medication side effects.
Examination	Conduct a focused physical examination, especially of gait and neurological signs; perform a mental status examination.	Identify parkinsonism and focal neurological deficits; identify psychiatric syndromes.
Rating scales	Perform formal bedside testing with SLUMS (Tariq et al. 2006), MoCA (Nasreddine et al. 2005), or comparable tool.	Determine severity of cognitive impairment, establish baseline, aid in diagnosis.
	Administer PHQ-9 (Spitzer et al. 1999) or GDS (Sheikh and Yesavage 1986), GAD-7 (Spitzer et al. 2006), AUDIT-C (Bush et al. 1998).	Screen for depression, anxiety, alcohol use.
Labs	Request plasma sodium, calcium, glomerular filtration rate (calculated), thyroid-stimulating hormone, vitamin B_{12}, liver function tests; if delirium suspected, obtain urinalysis.	Identify most common reversible causes of cognitive impairment.
	(optional) Request plasma FTA-ABS, HIV testing, plasma ammonia, blood glucose, pulse oximetry, thiamine level, pyridoxine level.	Rule out rarer causes of dementia.

TABLE 1–2. Practical assessment of dementia *(continued)*

What?	How?	Why?
Neuroimaging	Request structural neuroimaging with CT or MRI.	Assess extent of vascular disease; rule out NPH and SDH; identify focal atrophy (as in AD and FTD).
	(optional) Request functional neuroimaging with FDG-PET; DAT-SPECT.	Diagnose AD; differentiate AD and FTD; aid in diagnosis of LBD.
	Request amyloid PET and tau PET (not yet clinically available).	Diagnose AD.
Other optional assessments	Request neuropsychological testing.	Aid in diagnosis in complex situations, in younger patients, in patients with high premorbid intelligence.
	Request lumbar puncture.	Obtain AD biomarkers; aid in diagnosis of NPH; rule out CJD, neurosyphilis.
	Request polysomnography.	Rule out obstructive sleep apnea and REM sleep behavior disorder.
	Assess capacity (see Chapter 7).	Determine patient's capacity to make medical decisions and other decisions.

Note. AD = Alzheimer's disease; ADLs = activities of daily living; AUDIT-C = Alcohol Use Disorders Identification Test, consumption questions; BPSD = behavioral and psychological symptoms of dementia; CJD = Creutzfeldt-Jakob disease; CT = computed tomography; DAT-SPECT = dopamine transporter single-photon emission computed tomography; FDG-PET = fluorodeoxyglucose positron emission tomography; FTA-ABS = fluorescent treponemal antibody absorption; FTD = frontotemporal dementia; GAD-7 = Generalized Anxiety Disorder 7-item scale; GDS = Geriatric Depression Scale (short form); LBD = Lewy body disease; MoCA = Montreal Cognitive Assessment; MRI = magnetic resonance imaging; NPH = normal pressure hydrocephalus; PET = positron emission tomography; PHQ-9 = Patient Health Questionnaire–9; REM = rapid eye movement; SDH = subdural hematoma; SLUMS = Saint Louis University Mental Status examination.

scribed in much greater detail in Chapter 4, it is essential to ask the patient about BPSD—namely, depression, anxiety, irritability/anger, hallucinations, delusions, suicidal ideation, homicidal ideation, sleep disturbance, and aggression. The patient should then be asked about any functional impairments, as detailed earlier in the section "Background and Terminology," with close attention paid to problems with driving, cooking, ambulating, taking medications, or other aspects of self-care that could pose a threat to safety. Use of alcohol, caffeine, and illicit substances (amount, frequency, consequences) should be assessed; misuse of prescription medications should also be assessed. The person with dementia may become fatigued or frustrated with an extensive interview, so this part of the assessment may become more focused or conducted on separate occasions.

History From Informants

The clinician should also collect the information specified above from family members and other informants. It can be instructive to interview the patient and informant together. Because the histories may be different, I explain to the patient ahead of time that he or she and the informant may have different opinions, and it is important for me to hear all perspectives. If the patient has the capacity to give consent to have an informant present, then he or she should do so. Sometimes, however, this is simply too distressing for the patient (especially when discussing challenging behaviors), in which case the interviews should occur separately. Of course, if the clinician has any concern whatsoever about elder abuse (e.g., if the patient appears frightened, apprehensive, or withdrawn when with caregiver; appears malnourished; has cuts or bruises; or appears unkempt or disheveled), then the patient must be interviewed alone and screened for elder abuse; a tool such as the Elder Abuse Suspicion Index (EASI; Yaffe et al. 2008) may then be helpful (see the section "Screening for Elder Abuse" in Chapter 2 and the section "Protecting the Vulnerable Elder With Dementia" in Chapter 7 for further discussion, and see Table 2–3 in Chapter 2 for the EASI).

Chart Review

Data may come from various sources, such as the patient's medical record at the clinician's institution, the medical record at an outside institution, notes from the facility where the patient resides, notes from an informant, and a questionnaire completed by the patient or informant prior to the assessment (e.g., the Pre-evaluation Form in the Appendix to this book). The following are especially important to review: medication list, including over-the-counter medications, nutraceuticals, and complementary and alternative medicine treatments; past medical history; past psychiatric history; family history of neurological and psychiatric disorders, especially dementia; laboratory tests in the past year; any prior neuroimaging studies; prior neuropsychological testing; and any prior neurological, psychiatric, and geriatric evaluations. If the patient has already been found to not have capacity to make medical decisions, then the relevant paperwork (power of attorney or guardianship documents) should be reviewed.

Examination

The clinician should check vital signs and conduct a focused physical examination, targeting the neurological system. The mental status examination should include queries about mood, hallucinations, delusions, suicidal ideation, and homicidal ideation if such questions have not been previously asked. Appearance, behavior, affect, thought processes, insight, and judgment should be assessed. Level of arousal and orientation should be noted.

Rating Scales

The clinician should assess cognition using a bedside tool such as the SLUMS examination or the Montreal Cognitive Assessment (MoCA; Nasreddine et al. 2005). This will help the clinician determine the severity of cognitive impairment, will help to establish a baseline, and may aid in differential diagnosis, based on the pattern of responses. For example, significant trouble with the memory questions coupled with good performance on other questions could be consistent with AD. Other important assessments to consider include scales to assess depression (PHQ-9 [Spitzer et al. 1999] or Geriatric Depression Scale [GDS; Sheikh and Yesavage 1986], short form), anxiety (Generalized Anxiety Disorder 7-item scale [GAD-7; Spitzer et al. 2006]), and alcohol use (the consumption questions of the Alcohol Use Disorders Identification Test [AUDIT-C; Bush et al. 1998]).

Laboratory and Other Investigations

To rule out the most common reversible etiologies of dementia, the following tests are recommended: serum sodium, calcium, glomerular filtration rate (calculated based on creatinine, age, gender, ethnicity), thyroid-stimulating hormone, vitamin B_{12} level, and liver function tests (Rabins et al. 2007). If delirium is suspected, a urinalysis should be obtained to rule out a urinary tract infection. If other etiologies are suspected, additional lab tests can be ordered (Table 1–2).

Structural neuroimaging should be a standard part of assessing dementia, especially for patients with vascular risk factors, early onset (before age 65), or history or physical examination of a focal neurological lesion (Rabins et al. 2007). In most cases, CT should suffice: it is quick, tolerable to patients, and able to identify NPH, subdural hematoma, and significant cerebrovascular disease. MRI may be preferable to identify focal lobar atrophy (e.g., to aid in the diagnosis of AD or FTD) or to better delineate the location and extent of cerebrovascular disease. There may be some instances in which neuroimaging is not necessary, such as for a patient with a history very consistent with AD, no atypical features, a normal neurological examination, and normal basic laboratory testing.

Functional neuroimaging with FDG-PET may be helpful in the diagnosis of AD, in the diagnosis of DLB, or in distinguishing AD from FTD (Ahmed et al. 2014). FDG-PET measures metabolic activity within the brain: hypometabolism in temporal and parietal lobes is consistent with AD, hypometabolism in frontal or frontal and temporal lobes is consistent with FTD, and hypometabolism in the occipital lobe is consistent with DLB. Dopamine transporter SPECT (DAT-SPECT) could aid in the diagnosis of DLB. Although not yet clinically available or used, amyloid PET and tau PET may eventually allow for earlier and more accurate diagnosis of AD.

Neuropsychological testing yields a much more detailed cognitive assessment than what can be done at the bedside (Rabins et al. 2007). Results are reported for various cognitive domains (e.g., memory, language, visuospatial functioning) and in percentiles, controlling for age and educational background. Neuropsychological testing may be particularly useful in helping determine the diagnosis in patients with MCI or early dementia, in complex clinical situations, in patients with high premorbid intelligence (who may have false-negative bedside testing), and in patients whose first language differs from the language of the culture around them. Testing may also establish a baseline and identify domains of preserved cognition. The chief drawback is that someone with specific expertise (a neuropsychologist or a neuropsychologist working together with a psychometrist) must administer the tests.

Lumbar puncture can be used to obtain biomarkers for AD. Low levels of $A\beta_{42}$ or high levels of phosphorylated tau in cerebrospinal fluid are consistent with AD; this procedure is not part of routine clinical practice (Ahmed et al. 2014). Lumbar puncture can also be used to diagnose NPH (elevated opening pressure), to confirm neurosyphilis (following up on a positive serum treponemal test such as fluorescent treponemal antibody absorption [FTA-ABS]), and to confirm CJD (presence of 14-3-3 protein).

Polysomnography is indicated to rule out obstructive sleep apnea, a potentially reversible cause of cognitive impairment, and REM sleep behavior disorder, a condition suggestive of DLB (McKeith et al. 2017).

Genetic testing, including *APOE* genotyping, is very rarely part of a dementia evaluation. In suspected cases of autosomal dominant AD (very strong family history of early-onset dementia), testing for *PS1*, *PS2*, and *APP* mutations could be ordered (Rabins et al. 2007).

Making the Diagnosis

The following diagnostic criteria will aid the clinician in diagnosing the most common causes of dementia. (Also, see Table 1–1.)

- DSM-5 criteria for *major neurocognitive disorder due to AD* include 1) presence of major neurocognitive disorder (dementia); 2) insidious onset of symptoms; 3) decline in memory and at least one other cognitive domain; 4) progressive and gradual decline in cognition, without extended plateaus; and 5) no evidence of other etiologies (American Psychiatric Association 2013).
- Alternatively, the National Institute on Aging–Alzheimer's Association criteria for *probable AD dementia* include 1) presence of dementia; 2) insidious onset of symptoms; 3) worsening of symptoms, according to either the patient or observers; 4) initial and most prominent cognitive symptom being amnesia (usually the case in AD), word-finding deficits, visuospatial deficits, or executive dysfunction; and 5) absence of substantial cerebrovascular disease, features of DLB, and features of FTD (McKhann et al. 2011).
- The DLB Consortium criteria for *DLB* include 1) presence of dementia; 2) core clinical features of fluctuating cognition, recurrent visual hallucinations that are typically well formed and detailed, REM sleep behavior disorder (which may precede cognitive decline), and parkinsonism; and 3) supportive clinical features. Although not yet having widespread use outside of academic settings, the following studies could be ordered to support or rule out DLB: DAT-SPECT or PET; [123]iodine-MIBG myocardial scintigraphy; or polysomnography (especially in patients with history of REM sleep behavior disorder) (McKeith et al. 2017).
- Given the heterogeneity of vascular dementia, no one criterion set seems to have optimal sensitivity and specificity. The DSM-5 criteria for *major vascular neurocognitive disorder* include 1) presence of major neurocognitive disorder; 2) cognitive deficits that are temporally related to cerebrovascular events or are most notable in attention or executive function; and 3) evidence of cerebrovascular disease (e.g., as found on neuroimaging) (American Psychiatric Association 2013).
- International consensus criteria for the *behavioral variant of FTD* include 1) progressive deterioration of behavior and/or cognition; 2) functional decline; 3) neuroimaging findings of atrophy or hypometabolism in fron-

tal and/or anterior temporal lobes; and some combination of 4) early (within the first 3 years) behavioral disinhibition, 5) early apathy, 6) early loss of empathy, 7) early repetitive behaviors, and 8) hyperorality (Rascovsky et al. 2011).

One should strongly consider the possibility of delirium when there is 1) acute onset of cognitive impairment, 2) fluctuation of symptoms, 3) acute onset of behavioral and psychological symptoms, or 4) marked change from prior cognitive, behavioral, or psychological symptoms. Delirium is quite prevalent in patients with dementia and may in fact be when dementia is first identified. The Confusion Assessment Method operationalizes the DSM-III-R (American Psychiatric Association 1987) criteria for delirium (Inouye et al. 1990): the diagnosis of delirium requires the presence of 1) acute onset and fluctuating course and 2) inattention, and either 3) disorganized thinking or 4) altered level of consciousness (hyperalert, lethargic, obtunded, comatose). (See Figure 4–4.)

SUMMARY: PRACTICAL CONSIDERATIONS WHEN DIAGNOSING DEMENTIA

Every patient with cognitive impairment deserves a diagnosis—that is, identifying what the cause of his or her cognitive impairment is. When a patient presents acutely—with a delirium or with BPSD that require immediate attention—a comprehensive evaluation may need to be deferred. Obtaining a diagnosis helps patients and their families understand the disease and its prognosis, ensures that reversible etiologies are addressed, facilitates planning (in fact, this is one of the key advantages of an early diagnosis of dementia), and informs treatment planning (see Chapter 2).

The most common cause of dementia is AD, which can now be diagnosed fairly reliably and accurately; as researchers gain more understanding of the neuropathology of AD, medical professionals will be able to diagnose the disease earlier and even more accurately. An older patient (say, age 75 years or older) with progressive decline in memory and language, functional impairment, no atypical features, normal neurological examination, and a laboratory evaluation that has excluded common reversible causes, most likely has AD.

Other important causes of dementia to consider, especially in a patient presenting with BPSD, include DLB, PDD, vascular dementia, and FTD. Each of these has its own neuropsychiatric presentation, course, prognosis, and associated BPSD. When there is an acute onset of symptoms, fluctuation of symptoms, or a marked change in symptoms, delirium must be considered.

The assessment of a patient with suspected dementia should, at a minimum, include history from patient and other informants, review of records (especially use of medications and other substances), focused physical examination and mental status examination, and laboratory tests and neuroimaging targeted to the most likely diagnoses.

KEY POINTS

- An important step in understanding and addressing BPSD is diagnosing the cause of dementia. The presentation of BPSD varies by diagnosis, and the diagnosis may influence the treatment approach.
- The most common cause of dementia is AD, but clinicians should also be aware of vascular dementia, Lewy body disease, FTD, and mixed dementia. These conditions have differing presentations, prognoses, and treatments.
- The comprehensive assessment of dementia includes obtaining a history from the patient and informants (cognitive symptoms, BPSD, ADLs), thorough chart review (with an emphasis on medications, other substances, and past medical and psychiatric history), focused physical examination and mental status examination, bedside cognitive testing, and laboratory and imaging investigations tailored to suspected diagnoses.
- The evaluation of a person with cognitive impairment should include ruling out reversible causes, especially depression, hypothyroidism, medications, alcohol, vitamin B_{12} deficiency, and electrolyte disturbance.
- Atypical features, such as acute onset, rapid decline, young age, and the presence of neurological signs and symptoms, should lead to a more extensive evaluation.

RESOURCES FOR PATIENTS, FAMILIES, AND CAREGIVERS

Alzheimer's Association (www.alz.org) helps educate and support patients and their caregivers and also promotes research into AD. The organization hosts patient and caregiver education and support groups throughout the United States. The 24/7 helpline number is 800-272-3900.

Alzheimer's Disease International (www.alz.co.uk) is an international federation of Alzheimer's associations around the world. The website contains a wide range of educational information, including on clinical trials and on dementia-friendly communities.

The Association for Frontotemporal Dementia (www.theaftd.org) provides a wide range of educational resources and has a webinar series presented by experts in FTD.

Lewy Body Dementia Association (www.lbda.org) produces a monthly digest summarizing the latest news on DLB and PDD and provides links to support groups around the United States. Note that the Parkinson's Foundation (www.parkinson.org) and American Parkinson Disease Association (www.apdaparkinson.org) provide valuable resources, though perhaps more focused on the motor symptoms of PD.

National Institute on Aging (www.alzheimers.gov) is the U.S. government's portal to information on Alzheimer's disease and related dementias. The website includes the Alzheimer's and related Dementias Education and Referral Center (ADEAR). The resources are very comprehensive, including "Understanding Alzheimer's Disease: What You Need to Know" (available for download or a paper copy, both for free).

REFERENCES

Ahmed RM, Paterson RW, Warren JD, et al: Biomarkers in dementia: clinical utility and new directions. J Neurol Neurosurg Psychiatry 85(12):1426–1434, 2014 25261571

Alzheimer's Association: 2017 Alzheimer's disease facts and figures. Alzheimers Dement 13(4):325–373, 2017

American Psychiatric Association: Diagnostic and Statistical Manual of Mental Disorders, 3rd Edition, Revised. Washington, DC, American Psychiatric Association, 1987

American Psychiatric Association: Diagnostic and Statistical Manual of Mental Disorders, 5th Edition. Arlington, VA, American Psychiatric Association, 2013

Bang J, Spina S, Miller BL: Frontotemporal dementia. Lancet 386(10004):1672–1682, 2015 26595641

Bush K, Kivlahan DR, McDonell MB, et al: The AUDIT alcohol consumption questions (AUDIT-C): an effective brief screening test for problem drinking: Ambulatory Care Quality Improvement Project (ACQUIP): Alcohol Use Disorders Identification Test. Arch Intern Med 158(16):1789–1795, 1998 9738608

Charidimou A, Gang Q, Werring DJ: Sporadic cerebral amyloid angiopathy revisited: recent insights into pathophysiology and clinical spectrum. J Neurol Neurosurg Psychiatry 83(2):124–137, 2012 22056963

Clifford DB, Ances BM: HIV-associated neurocognitive disorder. Lancet Infect Dis 13(11):976–986, 2013 24156898

Dickson DW: Neuropathology of non-Alzheimer degenerative disorders. Int J Clin Exp Pathol 3(1):1–23, 2009 19918325

Dubois B, Feldman HH, Jacova C, et al: Research criteria for the diagnosis of Alzheimer's disease: revising the NINCDS-ADRDA criteria. Lancet Neurol 6(8):734–746, 2007 17616482

Ghanem KG: Review: neurosyphilis: a historical perspective and review. CNS Neurosci Ther 16(5):e157–e168, 2010 20626434

Glatzel M, Stoeck K, Seeger H, et al: Human prion diseases: molecular and clinical aspects. Arch Neurol 62(4):545–552, 2005 15824251

Harisingani R: Where are the reversible dementias? J Am Geriatr Soc 53(6):1066–1068, 2005 15935036

Inouye SK, van Dyck CH, Alessi CA, et al: Clarifying confusion: the Confusion Assessment Method: a new method for detection of delirium. Ann Intern Med 113(12):941–948, 1990 2240918

Jack CRJr, Bennett DA, Blennow K, et al: A/T/N: an unbiased descriptive classification scheme for Alzheimer disease biomarkers. Neurology 87(5):539–547, 2016 27371494

Katz S: Assessing self-maintenance: activities of daily living, mobility, and instrumental activities of daily living. J Am Geriatr Soc 31(12):721–727, 1983 6418786

Mayeda ER, Glymour NM, Quesenberry CP, Whitmer RA: Inequalities in dementia incidence between six racial and ethnic groups over 14 years. Alzheimers Dement 12(3):216-224, 2016 26874595

McGeer PL, McGeer EG: Inflammation, autotoxicity and Alzheimer disease. Neurobiol Aging 22(6):799–809, 2001 11754986

McKeith IG, Boeve BF, Dickson DW, et al: Diagnosis and management of dementia with Lewy bodies: fourth consensus report of the DLB Consortium. Neurology 89(1):88–100, 2017 28592453

McKhann GM, Knopman DS, Chertkow H, et al: The diagnosis of dementia due to Alzheimer's disease: recommendations from the National Institute on Aging–Alzheimer's Association workgroups on diagnostic guidelines for Alzheimer's disease. Alzheimers Dement 7(3):263–269, 2011 21514250

Nasreddine ZS, Phillips NA, Bédirian V, et al: The Montreal Cognitive Assessment, MoCA: a brief screening tool for mild cognitive impairment. J Am Geriatr Soc 53(4):695–699, 2005 15817019

O'Brien JT, Thomas A: Vascular dementia. Lancet 386(10004):1698–1706, 2015 26595643

Petersen RC, Roberts RO, Knopman DS, et al: Mild cognitive impairment: ten years later. Arch Neurol 66(12):1447–1455, 2009 20008648

Rabins PV, Blacker D, Rovner BW, et al: American Psychiatric Association practice guideline for the treatment of patients with Alzheimer's disease and other dementias, second edition. Am J Psychiatry 164 (12 suppl):5–56, 2007

Rascovsky K, Hodges JR, Knopman D, et al: Sensitivity of revised diagnostic criteria for the behavioural variant of frontotemporal dementia. Brain 134(Pt 9):2456–2477, 2011 21810890

Ridley NJ, Draper B, Withall A: Alcohol-related dementia: an update of the evidence. Alzheimers Res Ther 5(1):3, 2013 23347747

Sahyouni R, Goshtasbi K, Mahmoodi A, et al: Chronic subdural hematoma: a perspective on subdural membranes and dementia. World Neurosurg 108:954–958, 2017 28935547

Sheikh JI, Yesavage JA: Geriatric Depression Scale (GDS): Recent evidence and development of a shorter version. Clin Gerontol 5:165–173, 1986

Shprecher D, Schwalb J, Kurlan R: Normal pressure hydrocephalus: diagnosis and treatment. Curr Neurol Neurosci Rep 8(5):371–376, 2008 18713572

Sperling RA, Aisen PS, Beckett LA, et al: Toward defining the preclinical stages of Alzheimer's disease: recommendations from the National Institute on Aging–Alzheimer's Association workgroups on diagnostic guidelines for Alzheimer's disease. Alzheimers Dement 7(3):280–292, 2011 21514248

Spitzer RL, Kroenke K, William JR: Validation and utility of a self-report version of PRIME-MD: the PHQ primary care study: primary care evaluation of mental disorders: Patient Health Questionnaire. JAMA 282(18):1737–1744, 1999 10568646

Spitzer RL, Kroenke K, Williams JB, Löwe B: A brief measure for assessing generalized anxiety disorder: the GAD-7. Arch Intern Med 166(10):1092-1097, 2006 16717171

Suárez-González A, Henley SM, Walton J, et al: Posterior cortical atrophy: an atypical variant of Alzheimer disease. Psychiatr Clin North Am 38(2):211–220, 2015 25998111

Tariq SH, Tumosa N, Chibnall JT et al: Comparison of the Saint Louis University Mental Status examination and the Mini-Mental State Examination for detecting dementia and mild neurocognitive disorder—a pilot study. Am J Geriatr Psychiatry 14(11):900–910, 2006 17068312

University of Ottawa: Activities of Daily Living (ADL). Ottawa, Ontario, Canada, University of Ottawa, 2014. Available at: https://www.med.uottawa.ca/sim/data/Disability_ADL_e.htm. Accessed August 12, 2018.

Yaffe MJ, Wolfson C, Lithwick M, et al: Development and validation of a tool to improve physician identification of elder abuse: the Elder Abuse Suspicion Index (EASI). J Elder Abuse Negl 20(3):276–300, 2008 18928055

CHAPTER 2

COMPREHENSIVE MANAGEMENT OF DEMENTIA

Précis

A comprehensive plan to address dementia includes attempting to preserve cognition; educating and supporting family members and other caregivers; supporting activities of daily living (ADLs) with a goal of maintaining independence as long as possible; monitoring for and addressing safety issues; helping patients and their families plan for the future; and addressing behavioral and psychological symptoms of dementia (BPSD), the topic of the rest of this book. It is reasonable to consider a trial of a cognitive enhancer for any patient newly diagnosed with Alzheimer's disease (AD), Parkinson disease dementia (PDD), or dementia with Lewy bodies (DLB). All patients with dementia should avoid medications and substances that can have a negative effect on cognition, including alcohol. There may be some benefit to physical exercise, cognitive stimulation, and dietary changes. It is critical for clinicians to counsel and help support patients with dementia and their caregivers—fortunately, a wide variety of resources are available in the community, in print, and online.

EDUCATING AND SUPPORTING PATIENTS AND THEIR FAMILIES

The traditional medical relationship is between patient and clinician. For patients with dementia, the situation becomes more complex: Usually, at least one other person—a spouse or partner, child, other relative, or other

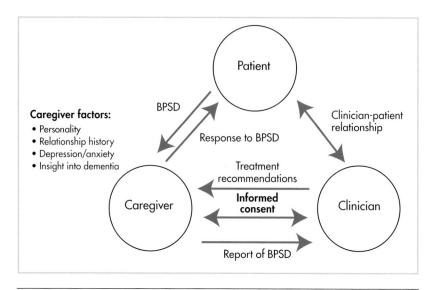

FIGURE 2–1.   The triad of patient, caregiver, and clinician.
BPSD=behavioral and psychological symptoms of dementia.

caregiver—is involved (Figure 2–1). Both the patient and the caregiver(s)
report symptoms to the clinician. A caregiver's report of symptoms may be
influenced by caregiver and relationship factors. The relationship between
the patient and a caregiver includes the patient's behavioral and psychological symptoms that may be directed toward the caregiver (e.g., aggression)
and the caregiver's response. If the patient does not have the capacity to
make medical decisions, a proxy decision maker must consent to the clinician's treatment recommendations. In many situations, more than one caregiver is involved, thus making these relationships even more complex.
Therefore, educating and supporting patients, families, and other caregivers
are critical.

Upon diagnosis of dementia, patients and their caregivers should be given
written information about the following: cause or causes of dementia, course
and prognosis, available treatments, and resources available for education and
support in the community, such as patient and caregiver support groups (National Institute for Health and Care Excellence 2006). The clinician may
recommend online or other written resources, such as *The 36-Hour Day* by
Mace and Rabins (2017). The clinician should also discuss with the patient
and family any support that is needed in the patient's home, identify and
address safety issues (e.g., cooking, driving), and help plan for the future
(see later sections of chapter for more details). Patients and families should

be informed of services available to provide support within the home, help with meals, and help with transportation and respite care. Patients and families may derive benefit from attending educational and support groups organized by the local chapter of the Alzheimer's Association and from talking with staff at their local area agency on aging, senior center, or aging and disability resource center.

The diagnosis of dementia may help explain to a patient and caregivers why the patient has been experiencing symptoms such as memory loss, repetitive questions and statements, word-finding difficulties, slowed responses, misplacing items, getting lost, having trouble with ADLs, and behavior changes. It may be useful and even necessary to explain to caregivers that the patient's actions are not volitional, manipulative, or targeted at caregivers but rather are symptoms of a brain disease. Tips for communicating with a patient with dementia include the following:

- Speak slowly, clearly, and directly to the patient.
- Give the patient adequate time to respond.
- Do not interrupt, correct, criticize, or argue.
- Break down questions, statements and requests into shorter phrases (e.g., replace a multiple-step request with a sequence of single-step requests).
- Give visual cues and demonstrations along with verbal statements.
- Use written notes as reminders and checklists.
- Be patient—easier said than done.

Individuals who care for patients with dementia are at risk of developing caregiver burnout, depression, and anxiety. Therefore, in addition to providing caregivers with education and support, clinicians should screen for depression and anxiety among caregivers and, if necessary, recommend more formal assessment and treatment. My own practice includes screening caregivers with an adaptation of the Patient Health Questionnaire–2 (PHQ-2; Löwe et al. 2005) by asking the following: "Over the last 2 weeks, have you felt down, depressed, or hopeless? Have you had little interest or pleasure in doing things?" If the caregiver answers "yes" to either one, I suggest that he or she contact his or her primary care provider for further assessment and treatment. I also recommend a caregiver support group and may refer the caregiver for individual psychotherapy.

Very few people can be patient and loving caregivers over sustained periods of time. Caregivers with certain personality structures may be especially challenged: those with narcissistic personality traits will find it difficult to be providers of care rather than recipients of attention and adulation; those with perfectionistic, rule-bound, and rigid personalities (i.e., obsessive-compulsive personality traits) may not have the flexibility and ability to "let go," which are very helpful when caring for someone with dementia; and those with avoidant or dependent personalities may not sufficiently advocate for themselves and their loved ones. Caregiving may also come toward the end of a decades-long relationship that, like all relationships, has had ups and downs—this is true of both marriages/partnerships and parent-child relationships. Preexisting disagreements, grudges, and grievances have a way of resurfacing under the strains of caregiving. Ensuring that caregivers have the support they need is therefore one of the most critical aspects of dementia care (National Institute for Health and Care Excellence 2006).

ENHANCING COGNITION

Someday a cure for AD and other causes of dementia will be found. When that day comes, the cognitive decline of dementia will be preventable and reversible. In the meantime, unfortunately, clinicians must make do with a short list of therapies that may delay, but not halt or reverse, cognitive decline. The strongest evidence is for acetylcholinesterase inhibitors and the N-methyl-D-aspartate (NMDA) antagonist memantine (Buckley and Salpeter 2015; National Institute for Health and Care Excellence 2011). Modest evidence exists for physical exercise and cognitive-enhancing strategies (McDermott et al. 2018) and perhaps dietary modifications (Singh et al. 2014; van de Rest et al. 2015). Almost all other pharmacological therapies, including initially very promising ones, have ultimately been found not to be effective (or, as in the case of estrogen, to be deleterious) (Cummings et al. 2014). Every effort should be made to discontinue medications (anticholinergic medications, benzodiazepines and other sedative-hypnotics, and opioids) and substances (alcohol and cannabis) that have negative effects on cognition. Most of the information presented in this section pertains to AD; other indications are noted as relevant.

Pharmacological Approaches

Currently, two classes of medications have been found to be modestly effective for delaying cognitive decline: *acetylcholinesterase inhibitors* and *NMDA antagonists*. Three acetylcholinesterase inhibitors—donepezil, rivastigmine, and galantamine—have been and remain approved for use in the United States and elsewhere (National Institute for Health and Care

Excellence 2011). The first drug in this class to be approved, tacrine, was subsequently withdrawn because of concerns about hepatoxicity (Buckley and Salpeter 2015). Since galantamine's approval in Sweden in 2000 (and other countries afterward), no other acetylcholinesterase inhibitors have been approved.

The mechanism of action of drugs in this class is to inhibit acetylcholinesterase, the enzyme that catalyzes the breakdown of acetylcholine, thereby making more acetylcholine available in the central nervous system (and also elsewhere, which is a cause of side effects). Patients with AD experience loss of cholinergic neurons, leading to decreased availability of acetylcholine as a neurotransmitter and, therefore, problems with attention and memory. Patients with DLB or PDD also experience cholinergic deficits, and this may also be the case in patients with vascular dementia. Rivastigmine also inhibits butyrylcholinesterase, which also hydrolyzes acetylcholine, but it is not clear what specific effect this inhibition has on rivastigmine's efficacy and tolerability.

As discussed in Chapter 1, disruption of the cholinergic system is a late step in the pathophysiology of AD. Increasing levels of acetylcholine are likely only to have a modest effect on the disease because earlier steps in abnormal amyloid and tau functioning are not altered. In fact, donepezil, rivastigmine, and galantamine appear to delay cognitive decline in patients with AD by about 6 months, after which time cognitive decline resumes. The cognitive and functional differences between drug-treated and placebo-treated patients may last up to 3 years, and there is some evidence that these drugs may delay placement in a nursing home (National Institute for Health and Care Excellence 2011).

Many patients cannot tolerate acetylcholinesterase inhibitors (Buckley and Salpeter 2015). An increase in cholinergic activity in the gastrointestinal system leads to nausea, vomiting, diarrhea, and loss of appetite, which can be especially problematic if a patient is frail or underweight to begin with. (In fact, discontinuation of acetylcholinesterase inhibitors has been associated with weight gain.) Parasympathetic effects in the cardiac system can lead to bradycardia, hypotension, dizziness, syncope, and falls; this is especially true when patients are also taking other prescribed agents that can cause bradycardia, such as β-blockers or centrally acting calcium channel blockers. Acetylcholine is quite active during rapid eye movement (REM) sleep, which may account for the side effects of insomnia and vivid dreams or nightmares. Finally, these medications can also cause muscle cramps and urinary incontinence. Side effects tend to arise early in treatment; slow titration is employed to reduce the risk of side effects. Contraindications to the use of acetylcholinesterase inhibitors include history of gastrointestinal ulcer or bleeding, uncontrolled asthma, angle-closure glaucoma, and problems with cardiac conduction (e.g., sick sinus syndrome, left bundle branch block) (Qaseem et al. 2008). Patients taking acetylcholinesterase inhibitors should not take medications with anticholinergic properties (e.g., medications to address urinary incontinence) at the same time because the latter will antagonize the effects of the former (Buckley and Salpeter 2015).

Head-to-head trials have not shown significant differences among the three approved acetylcholinesterase inhibitors (National Institute for Health and Care Excellence 2011). A high dosage (23 mg/day) of donepezil has been approved in the United States and elsewhere but appears to be associated with a marked increase in side effects without a comparable increase in benefit and therefore is rarely used (Knopman 2012). A patch version of rivastigmine bypasses first-pass metabolism, thereby resulting in fewer gastrointestinal side effects; however, patches themselves can be problematic on the frail skin of older adults, and they require rotation of application sites (which may need to be done by a caregiver). Donepezil is taken once a day, in the morning; oral rivastigmine is taken two times a day, whereas the patch is applied and removed each day; galantamine is available in both once-daily and twice-daily formulations. Dosing of galantamine must be adjusted in patients with renal impairment.

The only medication in the class of NMDA antagonists that has been found to be effective in treating AD is memantine. At first blush, it is not clear why a compound that blocks the glutamatergic NMDA receptor would aid cognition. Glutamate is a neurotransmitter critical for long-term potentiation, the molecular mechanism that underpins memory, and it acts at NMDA receptors. Phasic release of glutamate into synaptic clefts within the hippocampus is associated with memory formation. However, in AD it appears that there is excessive tonic (i.e., happening all of the time) release of glutamate, which is neurotoxic. Memantine appears to block the effects of the increased tonic levels of glutamate without interfering with the effects on NMDA of phasic release of glutamate; in other words, it may decrease neurotoxicity without negatively affecting memory (Buckley and Salpeter 2015).

Memantine offers modest benefit in delaying cognitive decline in patients with moderate to severe AD. Overall, memantine is well tolerated, with the most common side effects reported to be fatigue, increased blood pressure, dizziness, headache, constipation, confusion, and sleepiness; the risk of these side effects was not found to be higher in subjects who received memantine than in subjects who received placebo (Buckley and Salpeter 2015). Dosing of memantine must be adjusted in patients with renal impairment. After early enthusiasm that combining memantine and a cholinesterase inhibitor may be effective, subsequent analyses have not found added benefit from this combination (Buckley and Salpeter 2015; National Institute for Health and Care Excellence 2011). I argue that memantine's primary role is as an alternative when an acetylcholinesterase inhibitor is contraindicated, not tolerated, or clearly not effective. Table 2–1 summarizes the use of cognitive enhancers.

As noted earlier in this section, patients with DLB or PDD have cholinergic deficits, sometimes profound. Therefore, it would be reasonable to consider prescribing an acetylcholinesterase inhibitor to a patient with DLB or PDD; in fact, in the United States, rivastigmine is approved for use in PDD (Wang et al. 2015). Curiously, *anti*cholinergic medications have been used in the treatment of motor symptoms of Parkinson disease; however, these medications should be avoided if cognitive impairment is present.

The data supporting the use of acetylcholinesterase inhibitors and memantine for vascular dementia are quite weak, with a recent review concluding there was no evidence of efficacy (Baskys and Cheng 2012). No cognitive enhancers have been found to be effective in the treatment of cognitive symptoms of frontotemporal dementia (FTD). In the sole study of acetylcholinesterase inhibitors for FTD, galantamine did not improve cognition and may have caused agitation (Nardell and Tampi 2014; Young et al. 2018). In two studies of memantine, one did not find any benefit for FTD and the other raised concern that memantine could worsen cognition (Nardell and Tampi 2014; Young et al. 2018). Cognitive enhancers have not been shown to be effective in mild cognitive impairment (MCI).

There has been great controversy about the slim benefit afforded by acetylcholinesterase inhibitors and memantine and about whether the benefits outweigh the risks and costs associated with the medications. Although it is generally agreed that it is reasonable to prescribe an acetylcholinesterase inhibitor in mild or moderate stages of dementia due to AD as soon as the diagnosis is made, it is less clear what the latest point in disease course should be for starting a medication (though, at least in the United States, donepezil is approved for all stages of dementia due to AD, including severe dementia). Physicians are rarely able to determine in individual patients whether cognitive decline has been slowed. Family caregivers are often the best judges of such change. If a patient's cognition continues to decline at the same pace after starting an acetylcholinesterase inhibitor as it had been prior to starting it, the medication should be stopped; consideration could then

TABLE 2–1. Cognitive-enhancing medications

Medication	Dosing	Notes
Donepezil	5 mg/day at breakfast for 1 month, then 10 mg/day at breakfast thereafter	Contraindicated in patients with peptic ulcers, gastrointestinal bleeding, cardiac arrhythmias; most common side effects are nausea, vomiting, diarrhea, bradycardia, dizziness, syncope, falls, insomnia, nightmares, muscle cramps, urinary incontinence
Rivastigmine	Oral formulation: start 1.5 mg two times a day with meals, increase by 1.5 mg per dose every 2 weeks as tolerated, up to maximum of 6 mg two times a day[a] (titrate every 4 weeks in Parkinson disease dementia) Transdermal patch: 4.6-mg patch daily for 4 weeks, then 9.5-mg patch daily for 4 weeks, then 13.3-mg patch daily thereafter[a]	
Galantamine	Once-daily formulation: 8 mg at breakfast for 4 weeks, then 16 mg at breakfast for 4 weeks, then 24 mg at breakfast thereafter[a] Twice-daily formulation: 4 mg two times a day with meals for 4 weeks, then 8 mg two times a day for 4 weeks, then 12 mg two times a day thereafter[a]	
Memantine	Once-daily formulation: 7 mg/day for 1 week, then 14 mg/day for 1 week, then 21 mg/day for 1 week, then 28 mg/day thereafter Twice-daily formulation: 5 mg in morning for 1 week, then 5 mg two times a day for 1 week, then 10 mg in the morning and 5 mg at bedtime for 1 week, then 10 mg two times a day thereafter	Generally, well tolerated; alternative to acetylcholinesterase inhibitors when they are contraindicated or not tolerated; mixed evidence regarding efficacy when combined with donepezil

[a]Restart titration if interrupted for more than 3 days.

be given to prescribing memantine instead or, after a washout period so as to avoid excess cholinergic activity, another acetylcholinesterase inhibitor. If a patient is unable to tolerate an acetylcholinesterase inhibitor, that medication should be discontinued, and a trial of memantine could be considered.

It is unclear at what stage in the illness to stop these medications, and there has been some concern that cessation can lead to worsening of cognition, functioning, and behavior and perhaps even an increased risk of nursing home placement. It does not appear that cholinesterase inhibitors have an effect on survival (National Institute for Health and Care Excellence 2011). Some authors have recommended discontinuing a cognitive enhancer either when a patient enters the severe stage of dementia (though this contradicts the U.S. Food and Drug Administration approval for donepezil and memantine for severe dementia) or when a patient is institutionalized (Buckley and Salpeter 2015). Because there is a risk of withdrawal symptoms with sudden discontinuation of acetylcholinesterase inhibitors, the patient should be weaned from these medications, and the patient's clinical and functional status should be monitored closely. Ultimately, whether and when to stop a cognitive enhancer should be decided on an individual basis, weighing the possible benefits of long-term use and risks of discontinuation against the risks of continued use and the possibility that the medication is no longer of any benefit.

The National Health Service in the United Kingdom, after initially endorsing the use of acetylcholinesterase inhibitors, proposed in 2005 to no longer pay for them, citing doubts about their cost-effectiveness; after significant blowback, the National Health Service agreed to cover acetylcholinesterase inhibitors in some circumstances. If cognitive enhancers are cost-effective, it is due to a delay in institutionalization and the attendant reduction in costs offsetting the cost of the medications. The most recent guidelines of the National Institute for Health and Care Excellence in the United Kingdom state that donepezil, rivastigmine, and galantamine are options for the treatment of mild to moderate AD and that treatment "should be continued only when it is considered to be having a worthwhile effect on cognitive, global, functional or behavioural symptoms" (National Institute for Health and Care Excellence 2011). These guidelines list memantine as an option for patients with moderate AD who are intolerant of or who have a contraindication to acetylcholinesterase inhibitors and as an option for severe AD (National Institute for Health and Care Excellence 2011).

A quick note on the staging of dementia due to AD: There is not a universally agreed-upon way of determining if a patient has mild, moderate, or

FUNCTIONAL ASSESSMENT STAGING (FAST) (Check highest **consecutive** level of disability.)

1. **No difficulty**, either subjectively or objectively.

2. Complains of forgetting location of objects. **Subjective work difficulties.**

3. Decreased job functioning evident to co-workers. Difficulty in traveling to new locations. **Decreased organizational capacity.***

4. **Decreased ability to perform complex tasks**, e.g., planning dinner for guests, handling personal finances (such as forgetting to pay bills), difficulty marketing, etc.*

5. **Requires assistance in choosing proper clothing** to wear for the day, season, or occasion, e.g. patient may wear the same clothing repeatedly, unless supervised.*

6. (a) **Improperly putting on clothes without assistance or cuing** (e.g., may put street clothes on over night clothes, or put shoes on wrong feet, or have difficulty buttoning clothing) occasionally or more frequently over the past weeks.*

   (b) Unable to bathe properly (e.g., **difficulty adjusting bath-water temperature**) occasionally or more frequently over the past weeks.*

   (c) **Inability to handle mechanics of toileting** (e.g., forgets to flush the toilet, does not wipe properly or properly dispose of toilet tissue) occasionally or more frequently over the past weeks.*

   (d) **Urinary incontinence** (occasionally or more frequently over the past weeks).*

   (e) **Fecal incontinence** (occasionally or more frequently over the past weeks).*

7. (a) Ability to speak limited to approximately a **half a dozen intelligible different words or fewer**, in the course of an average day or **in the course of an intensive interview.**

   (b) Speech ability limited to the use of **a single intelligible word** in an average day or **in the course of an intensive interview** (the person may repeat the word over and over).

   (c) Ambulatory ability lost **(cannot walk without personal assistance).**

   (d) **Cannot sit up without assistance** (e.g., the individual **will fall over if there are no lateral rests** [arms] **on the chair).**

   (e) **Loss of ability to smile.**

   (f) **Loss of ability to hold up head independently.**

FIGURE 2–2. Staging of dementia: Functional Assessment Staging (FAST).

*Scored primarily on the basis of information obtained from a knowledgeable informant and/or caregiver.

Source. Reprinted from Reisberg B: "Functional Assessment Staging (FAST)." *Psychopharmacology Bulletin* 24:653–659, 1988. Copyright © 1984 by Barry Reisberg, M.D. Used with permission.

FUNCTIONAL ASSESSMENT STAGING (FAST)

INSTRUCTIONS

The **FAST Stage** is the highest consecutive level of disability. For clinical purposes, in addition to staging the level of disability, additional, non-ordinal (nonconsecutive) deficits should be noted, since these additional deficits are of clear clinical relevance.

For the purpose of therapeutic trials, the FAST can be used to sensitively encompass the full range in functional disability in CNS aging and dementia. For these purposes the **FAST Disability Score** should be obtained as follows:

(1) Each FAST substage should be converted into a numerical stage. Specifically, the following scoring should be applied: 6a = 6.0; 6b = 6.2; 6c = 6.4; 6d = 6.6; 6e = 6.8; 7a = 7.0; 7b = 7.2; 7c = 7.4; 7d = 7.6; 7e = 7.8; 7f = 8.0.

(2) The consecutive level of disability (FAST stage) is scored and given a numerical value.

(3) The nonconsecutive FAST deficits are scored. A nonconsecutive full stage deficit is scored as 1.0. A nonconsecutive substage deficit is scored as 0.2.

(4) The **FAST Disability Score** = (The FAST Stage Score) + (Each nonconsecutive FAST disability scored as described).

For example, if a patient is at FAST Stage 6a, then the patient's FAST stage score = 6.0. By definition, this patient cannot handle a job, manage their personal finances, independently pick out their clothing properly, or put on their clothing properly without assistance. If, in addition, this patient is incontinent of urine and cannot walk without assistance, then nonconsecutive deficits "6d" and "7c" are scored. The **FAST Disability Score** for this patient is 6.0 + 0.2 + 0.2 = 6.4.

FIGURE 2–2. Staging of dementia: Functional Assessment Staging (FAST) *(continued)*.

severe dementia. For example, in the National Institute for Health and Care Excellence (2011) guidelines, *mild* refers to Mini-Mental State Examination (MMSE; Folstein et al. 1975) scores of approximately 21–26, *moderate* 10–20, and *severe* 9 and below; slightly different cutoffs are used in different contexts. The MMSE, though a mainstay of research, is no longer in the public domain and free of charge, so it is now used less frequently in clinical settings, which limits applicability of these stages. The CDR (Clinical Dementia Rating; Morris 1993)—a registered trademark—is a dementia staging instrument, also used in research settings; CDR yields scores of 0.5 (MCI), 1 (mild dementia), 2 (moderate dementia), and 3 (severe dementia). CDR is discussed again in Chapter 6 in the context of addressing safety issues. Perhaps the most widely clinically accepted staging system is the Functional Assessment Staging (FAST) for AD, which finely delineates advanced dementia in particular. FAST and instructions for its use are detailed in Figure 2–2 (Reisberg 1988).

Unfortunately, many medications have been found to be ineffective at preventing or slowing cognitive decline in dementia. Between 2000 and 2012, of 413 clinical trials in AD, 99.6% were unsuccessful; of 244 compounds assessed, only one (memantine) was approved for clinical use (Cummings et al. 2014). As of the writing of this book, only four agents have been shown to have clear benefit in dementia, and this benefit is modest. Why are cognitive enhancers so minimally effective for cognitive impairment and—as discussed in Chapter 5—even less effective for BPSD? Cognitive enhancers do not act until a late step in the pathophysiological cascade that leads to dementia, which is essentially the end stage of a years-long neurodegenerative and cerebrovascular process. Interventions are needed that target earlier steps (e.g., in AD, the generation of toxic β-amyloid); developing such interventions will require earlier detection of the causes of dementia, specifically before cognitive impairment arises. Figure 2–3 summarizes the approach to addressing cognitive symptoms, including use of cognitive enhancers.

Psychosocial Approaches

Of the nonpharmacological approaches, physical exercise appears to have the most robust benefit for patients with dementia, with potential benefit for cognition, physical function (e.g., increased walking speed, decreased risk of falling, perhaps improved balance), and ADLs (McDermott et al. 2018). Exercise may also improve cognitive and physical outcomes in patients with Lewy body disease (Morrin et al. 2018). If exercise is effective, what kind should be recommended and how frequently should it be done?

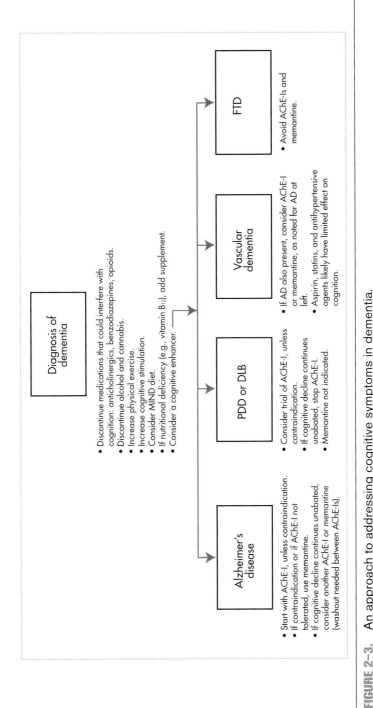

FIGURE 2–3. An approach to addressing cognitive symptoms in dementia.

AChE-I=acetylcholinesterase inhibitor; AD=Alzheimer's disease; DLB=dementia with Lewy bodies; FTD=frontotemporal dementia; MIND=Mediterranean-DASH Intervention for Neurodegenerative Delay (DASH=dietary approaches to stop hypertension); PDD=Parkinson disease dementia.

Studies of exercise use a wide variety of formats and frequencies, but it appears that exercise should take place at least twice weekly (and probably more than that) and for a total of at least 150 minutes per week per Centers for Disease Control and Prevention guidelines (2018 Physical Activity Guidelines Advisory Committee 2018). Exercise should include a variety of modalities, including walking, stretching, and strength training. There may be some benefit to exercising in a group, namely, socializing.

Anxious elders are the targets of the marketing of many "brain training" products, the majority of which have not been tested. Cognitive interventions include *cognitive stimulation*, which includes a range of activities to generally enhance cognition, often in a group format with an emphasis on social interaction and conducted by a trained therapist; *cognitive training*, which focuses on improving specific cognitive functions; and *cognitive rehabilitation*, in which patients develop their own goals and enact individualized approaches. Of the three, it appears that cognitive stimulation has the clearest benefit for cognition and may improve quality of life as well (McDermott et al. 2018). Cognitive training may benefit the specific cognitive domain in which training is taking place but does not appear to generalize to other cognitive domains.

Psychotherapy, which involves learning, cognitive processing, and reflection, can be challenging for patients with dementia. *Reminiscence therapy* is a form of psychotherapy in which patients discuss memories and past experiences, using photographs or music as prompts; reminiscence therapy may have slight benefit on cognition and quality of life (Woods et al. 2018). The role of psychosocial intervention is discussed in Chapter 5.

Vitamins, Diet, and Alcohol

The dietary habits of patients with dementia change as the disease evolves. Problems with smell (and therefore taste), memory loss, and executive dysfunction all may result in eating a less varied and lower-quality diet, may lead to weight loss, and might even cause or contribute to vitamin deficiencies. Patients with FTD may develop odd dietary habits, including eating nonfood items. If a patient with dementia is deficient in a vitamin known to be associated with cognition (B_1, B_6, B_{12}, or D), then the patient should take a prescribed supplement to address the deficiency. In patients without vitamin deficiencies, supplementation with vitamins does not appear to have an effect on cognition. Elevated homocysteine has been associated with dementia; though B-complex vitamins and folate lower homocysteine levels, this has not translated into cognitive benefits in patients with dementia (Zhang et al. 2017). Low levels of vitamin D may be prospectively associated with increased risk of dementia, but whether vitamin D supplementation mitigates this risk is unknown; the effect of correcting hypovitaminosis D on the risk of falls and fracture is also not entirely clear (Goodwill and Szoeke 2017). Opinions about the efficacy of vitamin E supplementation in dementia have varied over time. The most recent Cochrane review of four randomized placebo-controlled trials concluded that though subjects receiving vitamin E show less functional decline than those receiving placebo, vitamin E does not improve cognition in dementia and does not slow progression from MCI to AD (Farina et al. 2017). There has been concern about the safety of high-dose vitamin E supplements; however, this Cochrane review did not find an increased risk of death or other serious adverse events. I would not recommend routinely using vitamins in the treatment of dementia, except to address deficiencies in vitamins B_1, B_6, or B_{12}, and perhaps D.

A Mediterranean diet emphasizes vegetables and fruits, legumes, cereals, unsaturated fats (e.g., olive oil), and fish over meat, dairy, and saturated fats. Adhering to a Mediterranean diet may reduce the risk of developing MCI and AD and may slow the progression from MCI to AD. This conclusion is based on observational studies rather than prospective controlled trials (Singh et al. 2014). A prospective trial of the Mediterranean-DASH Intervention for Neurodegenerative Delay (MIND; DASH=dietary approaches to stop hypertension), which combines the Mediterranean diet with a low-sodium diet in patients who already have dementia, is under way (https://clinicaltrials.gov/ct2/show/NCT02817074). It would be reasonable to recommend that the patient with dementia (or whoever is preparing meals) implement some or all of the Mediterranean diet; though the benefits for cognition are not yet clear, there may be cardiovascular benefits and the risks are likely very low.

After early promise for omega-3 fatty acids, based on epidemiological data indicating lower incidence of dementia in those with higher dietary intake of omega-3 fatty acids, multiple studies have now demonstrated lack of efficacy in mild to moderate AD (Burckhardt et al. 2016). Omega-3 fatty acids at high doses are associated with a higher risk of bleeding. Furthermore, it has been suggested that a focus on the entire diet rather than on individual nutrients is more likely to be fruitful. Therefore, I would not recommend omega-3 fatty acid supplementation to address cognitive impairment in dementia.

Moderate use of alcohol (more than 0 and fewer than 30 g/day) is considered part of the Mediterranean diet and has been associated with a lower risk of developing dementia than abstinence and than higher levels of alcohol consumption (Piazza-Gardner et al. 2013). However, alcohol is also neurotoxic, with potentially negative effects on cognition, alertness, balance, and mood (Ridley et al. 2013). Therefore, once a patient has developed dementia, the risks of consuming alcohol likely outweigh the potential benefits, so alcohol use should be kept to a minimum or, if the top priority is preserving cognition, avoided entirely.

Complementary and Alternative Medicine

A variety of nutraceuticals have been tested in the treatment of AD, including ginkgo biloba (specifically, the extract EGb 761), curcumin, and huperzine A. Of these, the evidence seems to be strongest for ginkgo biloba; however, the most recent Cochrane review found methodological problems in studies of ginkgo biloba and concluded that the evidence for its efficacy is inconsistent and unreliable (Birks and Grimley Evans 2009). There is not enough evidence to support the use of curcumin or huperzine A in the treatment of dementia. Many other substances have been touted as having cognitive effects (e.g., apoaequorin, marketed in the United States as Prevagen, which does not survive digestion and does not cross the blood-brain barrier) without evidence supporting such claims. I would not recommend the use of any nutraceutical agents in the treatment of dementia.

ASSESSING AND SUPPORTING ACTIVITIES OF DAILY LIVING

A hallmark of dementia is impairment in ADLs. Typically, a patient with dementia first develops problems with instrumental ADLs, such as driving and money management, and then eventually progresses to having problems with personal ADLs, such as walking and toileting. (See the section on "Background and Terminology" in Chapter 1 for a full list of instrumental and personal ADLs.) A comprehensive dementia care plan includes an assessment of the current state of ADLs to determine which ADLs the patient can perform on his or her own, which ADLs the patient needs help with and has adequate help to do, and which ADLs the patient needs help with and lacks adequate help. Many of these ADLs are linked with safety issues, as described later and detailed in Chapter 6. Note that this assessment needs to be repeated over time as the disease progresses.

The care plan should include steps to support each of the ADLs, with a goal of maintaining the patient's independence as long as feasible. This topic is introduced here, and Chapter 6 focuses more on addressing associated safety concerns.

1. *Transportation:* One of the earliest abilities that people with AD lose is driving safely, which in turn affects their ability to conduct their affairs. Driving is a complex cognitive task that requires attention, memory, visuospatial function, and executive function to be intact and coordinated; patients with MCI even have an increased risk of motor vehicle accidents (Rabins et al. 2007). A sign of problems with driving may include getting lost even on familiar routes. Screening for driving safety is part of the joint American Academy of Neurology and American Psychiatric Association dementia management quality measures (Sanders et al. 2017). See Chapter 6 for further discussion of addressing driving safety. Installing GPS in the car might be helpful but does require learning a complex technology; encourage patients to keep their cell phones with them so they can call for help if they get lost. When a patient is no longer able to drive safely, alternative arrangements for transportation should be made. These include asking family members or friends to drive, using a taxi or ride-share service, and using special transportation services for older adults. Caregivers can reduce the need for transportation by arranging for delivery of medications, groceries, and meals.

2. *Finances:* Even fairly early in the course of dementia, patients develop problems with managing their finances, including paying bills. They may also become victims of exploitation (e.g., via phone scams) (Rabins et al. 2007). Arranging for a durable power of attorney (POA) of finances is recommended, preferably very early in the course of illness when the patient has more ability to understand this process and select his or her agent. Automatic bill paying services will ensure that bills are paid on time. In more extreme situations, guardianship may be necessary to ensure financial safety. See Chapters 6 and 7 for further discussion of financial exploitation and abuse.

3. *Food preparation:* Owing to memory loss, loss of sense of smell and taste, and decreased executive function, patients with dementia may have less ability to prepare meals. Safety can become a concern, too, such as when a patient puts unsafe items into a microwave or does not turn off a stove. Options to aid patients include having caregivers take over cooking, having meals delivered to the homes of older adults (e.g., Meals on Wheels), and arranging for congregate dining. See Chapter 6 for further discussion.

4. *Housekeeping:* Family members may need to take housekeeping responsibilities or hire housekeepers. Patients in assisted living facilities should be able to purchase housekeeping services. Chapter 6 covers other potential risks in the household, including access to firearms.

5. *Telephone:* Sensory, motor, and cognitive impairments may interfere with using a telephone, which in turn could lead to safety problems (not being able to call someone for help) or isolation and loneliness. Patients with dementia may benefit from simplified phones with large buttons, easy-to-read screens, and quick access to emergency services.

6. *Medications:* A critical first step for a clinician and patient is medication reconciliation: patients, family members, pharmacies, and electronic medical records may all have different accounts of what medications the patient is taking. This task also requires getting a complete list of over-the-counter and nutraceutical medications. The clinician should use this opportunity to carefully review all medications and eliminate those whose benefits do not outweigh risks (see discussion in the previous section). Patients with dementia may misuse medications by missing doses or taking extra doses or both. Options to ensure that patients take their medications appropriately include having family members set up weekly pill boxes; having family members monitor patients taking their medications; hiring an in-home service (e.g., visiting nurse) to monitor patients taking medications or to administer medications; having a pharmacy deliver weekly supplies of medications in pill boxes or blister packs; implementing automated reminders to take medications; and locking up medications when not in use. Patients in assisted living facilities should be able to purchase services to ensure that they are taking medications properly. See Chapter 6 for further discussion of medication safety.

7. *Ambulation:* Patients with dementia may have many risk factors for falling, in addition to dementia itself. These include vision loss, neuropathy, parkinsonism, medications, alcohol use, depression, malnutrition, dehydration, and deconditioning (Burton et al. 2015). Frequent falls are among the more common reasons for institutionalization of patients with dementia. Physical therapy may help address some of these concerns and lead to improved strength and balance as well as a recommendation for assistive devices. Electronic bracelets or pendants linked to emergency services may be useful, but they do require patients to remember that they have such a device and how to use it. See Chapter 6 for further discussion of assessing and addressing risk of falls.

8. *Toileting:* Urinary incontinence is not uncommon in older adults, and impairments in memory and mobility can compound this problem. Patients may become embarrassed, may avoid social situations and leaving the home, may develop problems with hygiene, and may be

prescribed anticholinergic medications with cognitive side effects. A medical evaluation may be necessary to identify a cause of urinary incontinence (e.g., recurrent urinary tract infections, benign prostatic hypertrophy, neuropathy) and fecal incontinence (e.g., bowel obstruction, chronic constipation, rectal prolapse). Strategies to address incontinence include regular toileting (especially at bedtime), using incontinence products (padded undergarments or adult briefs, incontinence pads on the bed, waterproof mattress covers), installing grab bars next to the toilet, or using a portable commode in the bedroom.

9. *Dressing and hygiene:* Patients with dementia may need prompts and assistance with personal care, with selecting clothes, and with putting on and taking off clothes. Either family members or hired in-home caregivers may assist with these tasks. This must be done with sensitivity to the patient's privacy and dignity.

10. *Eating:* Patients with dementia may eventually need reminders and cues to start and end meals. In advanced dementia, patients may have problems with chewing and swallowing, leading to complications such as aspiration pneumonia, a common cause of death in patients with dementia. Patients with dysphagia may need changes in their diet to reduce the risk of choking and aspiration. They may eventually need assistance with eating itself.

Clinicians should not underestimate the psychological impact of losing the ability to care for oneself. Patients with dementia may lack insight into their deficits, and the defense mechanism of denial (on the part of patients or their family members or both) may further complicate matters. Being told that one is no longer able to perform a task accomplished for decades (e.g., driving) can have a profound psychological effect—a threat to one's sense of self and dignity. A tension may arise between the ethical imperatives to respect a person's autonomy and to ensure that he or she is safe, and caregivers and clinicians must continually reassess the balance. Case Example 2–1 covers these issues and others described earlier.

Case Example 2–1: "How Can We Help Keep Mom at Home as Long as Possible?"

Mrs. Lewicki is a 79-year-old widow who was diagnosed 3 years ago with dementia due to AD. She has experienced memory loss, word-finding difficulties, occasional disorientation, and anxiety. She lives in a one-bedroom apartment in a senior living complex. She has hired a housekeeper who comes once a week, and her two adult children take turns checking in on her on the weekend. She is alone on weekdays and tends to watch a fair amount of television. She was advised to stop driving, so her children take her on errands and out to eat. After two incidents involving leaving food cooking on the stove, she now has one meal delivered to her each day; her other meals are simple, involving cereal, sandwiches, and ice cream. As best as her children can tell, she is taking her medications correctly: donepezil 10 mg/day, citalopram 20 mg/day, simvastatin 20 mg/day, lisinopril 5 mg/day, a multivitamin, acetaminophen as needed for back pain, and an over-the-counter "memory booster" she once saw advertised on television. She has two glasses of wine before bedtime; she does not smoke. She sees her primary care provider regularly; her blood pressure and cholesterol have been well controlled; a clinic social worker recently screened for elder abuse and did not find any evidence. Her family is not aware of any impairments other than the ones just described. They would like to honor Mrs. Lewicki's wish to live independently, so they ask her primary care provider, "How can we help keep Mom at home as long as possible?"

Mrs. Lewicki is already taking a cholinesterase inhibitor; memantine could be added to further delay cognitive and functional decline, though the evidence is mixed about the efficacy of such a combination. Her over-the-counter "memory booster" is unlikely to be helpful and should be discontinued. She is drinking alcohol in excess of the recommended amount for older adults; given that she already has cognitive impairment, it would be safest for her to cease drinking alcohol, both with respect to cognition and her risk of falls. Increasing her cognitive stimulation may be helpful, for example by participating in activities at her local senior center. It is unclear if she is exercising regularly; if not, this should be added to her routine. Her diet could be improved, specifically by reducing intake of ice cream and increasing intake of fruits, vegetables, and other elements of the MIND diet.

Her family should continue to monitor her ADLs. Given the concerns about cooking safety, she should consider disconnecting her stove. Her family should monitor her ability to manage her finances and especially be alert for any evidence that she may become a victim of a financial scam. If there any guns or power tools in the home, these should be removed. If she is not doing so already, she should arrange her medications in a weekly pill organizer or get help doing so. She and her family should ensure that she is still able to use her telephone to reach others and especially to get help.

If Mrs. Lewicki has not yet done so, she should execute a health care POA, financial POA, advance medical directive, and last will and testament. She and her family should have a frank and thorough discussion about her wishes for the future, including housing and medical care.

ADDRESSING SAFETY ISSUES

As dementia progresses, the risk of accidental harm increases. In the prior section, I discussed motor vehicle accidents, medication errors, problems with cooking, and falls, and I also address safety in Chapter 6. Other safety concerns include the following:

- Patients who smoke may accidentally cause a fire; cigarettes, matches, lighters, and ashtrays should be removed from sight, which may reduce the risk of fire as well as decrease cues to smoke.
- Wandering is common among patients with dementia and can lead to serious injury (e.g., falls, exposure) or death (Rabins et al. 2007). In some cases, the wandering is so frequent or dangerous that patients cannot be left alone. Strategies to help address wandering include installing alarms on doors; placing the patient on a local registry of people with dementia; having the patient wear an identification bracelet with the contact information of a caregiver; and having the patient wear a device to allow family members to track him or her. This topic is discussed in greater detail in Chapter 5.
- Family members should be instructed to remove guns from the home; if family members insist on keeping guns at home, the guns should be kept locked up, trigger locks installed, and ammunition kept separate. This is especially true for patients with suicidal ideation, a history of self-harm, or paranoia. The risk of suicide appears to be slightly elevated soon after the patient receives a diagnosis of dementia. The risk then declines, presumably due to executive dysfunction. Nevertheless, the risk of suicide among older adults is usually not zero, so caregivers and clinicians must take suicidal statements seriously.
- Patients with physical aggression may harm others or themselves. Much of Chapter 5 is devoted to nonpharmacological and pharmacological strategies to address agitation and aggression.

IDENTIFYING AND ADDRESSING PAIN

Older adults are at high risk of having chronic pain. For example, at least half of older adults have osteoarthritis; many have neuropathy, previous fractures, cancer, wounds (e.g., decubiti), or other musculoskeletal conditions (American Geriatrics Society Panel on Pharmacological Management of Persistent Pain in Older Persons 2009). About 64% of community-dwelling elders with dementia report pain that is bothersome, and 43% report pain that limits their activities (Hunt et al. 2015). On the other hand, some older adults with dementia (especially those with advanced dementia and those living in institutional settings) may have a hard time letting others know about their pain; with these patients, pain may manifest as withdrawal from physical and social activities, irritability, anxiety, insomnia, verbal aggression, physical aggression, or resistance to help with ADLs (e.g., dressing, bathing) (Hunt et al. 2015).

When a patient with dementia has unexplained changes in behavior or shows other signs of distress, he or she should be assessed for pain (American Geriatrics Society Panel on Pharmacological Management of Persistent Pain in Older Persons 2009). The most recent update to the joint American Academy of Neurology and American Psychiatric Association dementia management quality measures (which may be incorporated into Medicare's reimbursement system) includes the frequency with which clinicians screen for pain at all appointments with patients with dementia and, when pain is present, document a follow-up plan (Sanders et al. 2017). Patients with mild and moderate dementia may be screened for pain using a 0–10 numerical rating scale or a verbal descriptor scale such as the Revised Iowa Pain Thermometer (Ware et al. 2015; viewable online at www.painmanagementnursing.org/article/S1524-9042(14)00151-9/pdf). Interestingly, a visual analogue scale does not appear to be as reliable in older adults as a numerical or verbal scale. In patients with severe dementia, an observer-rated instrument such as the Pain Assessment in Advanced Dementia (PAINAD) scale may be helpful (Table 2–2) (Warden et al. 2003).

Addressing pain will depend on the underlying cause. For example, abdominal pain due to constipation should be addressed accordingly. In most other cases, analgesic medications should help reduce BPSD (Tampi et al. 2017). Treatment with scheduled acetaminophen 500–1,000 mg two or three times a day (up to a maximum of 3,000 mg/day) can be helpful (American Geriatrics Society Panel on Pharmacological Management of Persistent Pain in Older Persons 2009). Patients with hepatic disease or current alcohol use should avoid acetaminophen. A stepped protocol based on the American Geriatrics Society Panel on Pharmacological Management of Persistent Pain in Older Persons (2009) recommendations for treating pain in older adults has been found to reduce BPSD: acetaminophen up to 3,000 mg/day, extended-release oral morphine up to 20 mg/day, pregabalin up to 300 mg/day, or (for patients with swallowing difficulties) buprenorphine transdermal patch (Husebo et al. 2014).

Except in patients with hepatic disease or those who are still drinking alcohol, I routinely recommend scheduled acetaminophen starting at 1,000 mg two times a day and increasing to 1,000 mg three times a day for chronic pain. When patients and family members express skepticism about the effectiveness of acetaminophen, I note that scheduled administration resulting in a steady blood level of medication is more likely to be effective than "chasing pain" with as-needed doses. I personally feel less comfortable prescribing pre-

TABLE 2–2. Assessing pain in dementia: the Pain Assessment in Advanced Dementia (PAINAD) scale

Behavior	0	1	2
Breathing, independent of vocalization	Normal	Occasional labored breathing, short period of hyperventilation	Noisy labored breathing, long period of hyperventilation, Cheyne-Stokes respirations
Negative vocalization	None	Occasional moan or groan, low-level speech with a negative or disapproving quality[a]	Repeated troubled calling out, loud moaning or groaning, crying
Facial expression	Smiling or inexpressive	Sad, frightened, frowning	Grimacing
Body language	Relaxed	Tense, distressed pacing, fidgeting	Rigid, fists clenched, knees pulled up, pulling or pushing away, striking out
Consolability	No need to be consoled	Distracted or reassured by voice or touch	Unable to be consoled, distracted, or reassured

Note.   The clinician observes the patient for 5 minutes and then scores pain-related behaviors using the PAINAD on a 0–10 scale. Scores of 1–3 indicate mild pain, 4–6 moderate pain, and 7–10 severe pain.

[a]"Low-level speech with a negative or disapproving quality" refers to "muttering, mumbling, whining, grumbling, or swearing in a low volume with complaining, sarcastic, or caustic tone."

Source.   Reprinted from Warden V, Hurley AC, Volicer L: "Development and Psychometric Evaluation of the Pain Assessment in Advanced Dementia (PAINAD) Scale." *Journal of the American Medical Directors Association* 4(1): 9–15, 2003. Copyright 2003, with permission from Elsevier.

gabalin (due to cognitive side effects and risk of falls) and much less comfortable with opioids (though I have seen these to be helpful in patients with very advanced dementia and BPSD).

Other symptoms that clinicians should consider screening for and addressing are hearing loss, vision loss, nausea, dyspepsia, and constipation.

SCREENING FOR ELDER ABUSE

About 11% of older adults are victims of elder abuse, and the prevalence may be as high as 62% among those with dementia (Dong et al. 2014). Elder abuse includes physical abuse, sexual abuse, emotional or psychological abuse, neglect (including self-neglect, the most common type of elder abuse reported to state agencies), and financial abuse or exploitation. Elder abuse can occur at home or in a long-term care facility. In addition to dementia, risk factors for being abused include female sex, lower income, social isolation, being African American or Hispanic, having functional impairment or poor physical health, and manifesting BPSD (including aggression and depression) (Alosa Health 2017; Dong et al. 2014). Risk factors for perpetrating elder abuse include having a high perceived burden of care, abusing drugs or alcohol, having poor coping skills or low self-esteem, feeling levels of stress, experiencing depression or anxiety, being socially isolated, having cognitive impairment, having been abused oneself, and having had a poor relationship with the victim prior to the onset of dementia (Dong et al. 2014). Among caregivers of community-dwelling older adults, 26% reported that they had yelled or screamed at the recipient of care, and 18% reported that they had used a harsh tone, insulted, or sworn at the care recipient (Alosa Health 2017). Among the staff of long-term care facilities, risk factors include burnout and lower levels of job satisfaction (Dong et al. 2014).

Elder abuse can be lethal: the risk of death is three times higher among older adults suspected of being abused than among older adults not thought to be abused (Alosa Health 2017). Other consequences include disability, increased medical utilization, and greater risk of institutionalization (Alosa Health 2017).

Many cases of elder abuse are not detected. A number of screening tools are available, such as the Elder Abuse Suspicion Index (EASI), which has a sensitivity of 47% and specificity of 75% in detecting elder abuse in patients with an MMSE score of 24 or greater in ambulatory care settings (Yaffe et al. 2008; see Table 2–3). A "yes" response on one or more of questions 2–6 raises the possibility of elder abuse. The EASI is also available in Chinese, Estonian, Finnish, French, German, Greek, Hebrew, Italian, Japanese, Latvian, Nepali, Portuguese, Romanian, Spanish, and Turkish (McGill Department of Family Medicine 2018).

Rules for reporting elder abuse vary across jurisdictions. In the United States, local or state health departments have adult protective services programs, which investigate reports of abuse in the community, and long-term care ombudsman programs, which investigate reports of abuse in long-term

---

TABLE 2–3. Elder Abuse Suspicion Index

Clinician asks the patient the following questions regarding the last 12 months:

1. Have you relied on people for any of the following: bathing, dressing, shopping, banking, or meals?

2. Has anyone prevented you from getting food, clothes, medication, glasses, hearing aids or medical care, or from being with people you wanted to be with?

3. Have you been upset because someone talked to you in a way that made you feel shamed or threatened?

4. Has anyone tried to force you to sign papers or to use your money against your will?

5. Has anyone made you afraid, touched you in ways that you did not want, or hurt you physically?

Clinician answers the following question:

6. Elder abuse *may* be associated with findings such as poor eye contact, withdrawn nature, malnourishment, hygiene issues, cuts, bruises, inappropriate clothing, or medication compliance issues. Did you notice any of these today or in the last 12 months?

A "yes" response on one or more of questions 2–6 raises the possibility of elder abuse.

Source. © The Elder Abuse Suspicion Index (EASI) was granted copyright by the Canadian Intellectual Property Office (Industry Canada) February 21, 2006. (Registration No. 10364590). Used with permission.

---

care facilities. If a patient is in immediate danger, local law enforcement must be notified. Complicating matters is that patients with dementia may not have the capacity to agree to (or refuse) an investigation for elder abuse; furthermore, they may be unwilling to participate out of fear of retribution or loss of a caregiver; finally, the patients may have the capacity to refuse an investigation, leaving clinicians in an ethical quandary of whether to override the refusal and report anyway. There are few studies demonstrating how to effectively address elder abuse, although interventions aimed at addressing depression, anxiety, alcohol use, and poor coping strategies among caregivers may have promise, and increasing support and respite may also be helpful.

Clinicians should familiarize themselves with local regulations and laws regarding elder abuse, should maintain a high index of suspicion for elder abuse among their patients with dementia and screen accordingly, and must (with rare exceptions) report elder abuse to the appropriate local authorities. See the section "Financial Incapacity and Risk of Exploitation" in

Chapter 6 for a more detailed discussion of financial abuse and exploitation, and the section "Protecting the Vulnerable Elder With Dementia" in Chapter 7 for discussion of self-neglect, neglect, and abuse.

PLANNING FOR THE FUTURE AND LEGAL CONSIDERATIONS

One of the strongest arguments for the early diagnosis of dementia is that patients in the mild stage of dementia are more likely to be able to plan ahead and express their preferences for their care in the future than are patients in more severe stages (Rabins et al. 2007). Planning ahead may involve preparing the following documents:

- *Health care POA:* Selecting an agent to make medical decisions on behalf of the patient, in the event that the patient is no longer able to make such decisions
- *Financial POA:* Selecting an agent to help make financial decisions on behalf of the patient (may become active once a patient signs the document)
- *Advance directive or "living will":* Expressing wishes about future care, such as cardiopulmonary resuscitation (CPR), mechanical ventilation, and nursing home placement
- *Do not resuscitate (DNR) order:* Instructing health care providers to not administer CPR
- *Last will and testament:* Expressing wishes about what is to happen to one's assets and estate after death

When a patient is in more advanced stages of dementia, a clinician may need to assess the patient's capacity to execute one or more of these plans. A patient may retain an attorney to help prepare these documents; this process can be expensive, and there may be local legal services available, such as through the area agency on aging or through an aging and disability resource center.

Although the goal of most patients is to stay in their own homes, this is not always feasible. Planning for alternate housing in an assisted living facility, senior community, or skilled nursing facility can be a daunting process. It can be difficult to compare options, determine the costs, learn about how Medicare and Medicaid factor into costs, and identify resources available to defray costs. Terminology can be confusing: an *assisted living facility* can offer a wide range of services but typically not skilled nursing; *memory care units* purport to provide specialized services for patients with dementia, but they are not federally regulated and there appear to be no consensus criteria for what constitutes "memory care"; and *skilled nursing facilities* care for patients who require assistance with medications, toileting, or ambulation. I recommend referring patients and their families to their local agencies for assistance.

ADDRESSING BEHAVIORAL AND PSYCHOLOGICAL SYMPTOMS OF DEMENTIA

BPSD are the primary topic of this book. Ninety percent of patients with dementia experience BPSD at some point during their illness (Kales et al. 2014). These symptoms include depression, anxiety, irritability, paranoia, hallucinations, verbal aggression, physical aggression, apathy, and disturbances of the sleep-wake cycle. They result in reduced quality of life for both patients and caregivers, increased caregiver burden, increased risk of elder abuse, increased economic costs, and increased rates of institutionalization. I discuss how BPSD arise in Chapter 3, how to assess BPSD in Chapter 4, and how to manage BPSD in Chapter 5.

SUMMARY: DEVELOPING A COMPREHENSIVE PLAN TO MANAGE DEMENTIA

Dementia affects many facets of life: cognitive abilities, day-to-day functioning, emotions, relationships with others, and sense of self. Not surprisingly, treatment of dementia also encompasses many facets. The dementia care plan of all patients with dementia should include all of the elements listed in Table 2–4. I recommend that each objective be addressed upon initial assessment of a patient and then at least annually afterward. The Pre-evaluation Form (to be completed by the patient or a family member) provided in the Appendix may aid this process.

A person with dementia is no less a human being than one without dementia. Clinicians must support the person's autonomy, dignity, and sense of self-worth.

TABLE 2–4. A comprehensive plan to address dementia

Objective	Strategy
Teaching patients and family members about the illness and supporting them over the course of the illness	A number of resources are available, including in the community, in print, and online (see "Resources for Patients, Families, and Caregivers" section of each chapter in this book).
Addressing the needs of caregivers	Rates of depression and anxiety are high among caregivers, and their relationship with the recipients of their care will change over time. Caregivers should be screened for depression and referred appropriately.
Trying to preserve memory and delay cognitive decline	Options include donepezil, rivastigmine, galantamine, memantine (alone or in combination with donepezil), limiting alcohol use, eliminating medications that hamper cognition, physical exercise, cognitive stimulation, and (perhaps) dietary changes.
Supporting activities of daily living (ADLs) and helping patients attain their goals with respect to independence and housing	This objective requires an initial comprehensive assessment of ADLs and a recommendation for ways of supporting ADLs. Because dementia is progressive, this assessment will need to be repeated over time, at least annually.
Considering pain and other physical symptoms that could affect quality of life and behavior	Pain is underrecognized in patients with dementia; scheduled acetaminophen may an effective treatment. Also, clinicians should screen for and address hearing loss, vision loss, nausea, dyspepsia, and constipation.
Ensuring a safe environment, including one free of abuse and neglect	Impairments in memory, attention, and judgment can lead to problems with driving, taking medications correctly, cooking, and wandering. All of these must be monitored and addressed. Alternatives to driving should be recommended and eventually required. Clinicians should screen for problems with driving, falls, fire safety, and firearm safety at least annually. Screening for and addressing elder abuse should take place at baseline and whenever concern arises.

TABLE 2–4. A comprehensive plan to address dementia *(continued)*

Objective	Strategy
Planning ahead to a time when one may not be able to make their own medical, personal, and financial decisions	This planning is part of the rationale for early diagnosis of dementia. Planning ahead includes one or more of the following: health care power of attorney, financial power of attorney, advance directives, do-not-resuscitate order, and a will.
Addressing behavioral and psychological symptoms of dementia (BPSD)	Patients should be screened for BPSD, with caregivers also serving as informants (see Chapter 4 for more details). Nonpharmacological treatment should be a priority, with pharmacological treatment reserved for situations wherein safety is threatened or there is severe distress (see Chapter 5).

KEY POINTS

- Upon diagnosis of dementia, patients and their caregivers should be given written information about the following: cause or causes of dementia, course and prognosis, available treatments, and resources available for education and support in the community and online.

- Dementia caregivers are at risk of developing caregiver burnout, depression, and anxiety. Therefore, they should be screened and referred for treatment.

- There are limited options for addressing cognitive impairment:

  - The benefits of cognitive enhancers (donepezil, rivastigmine, galantamine, memantine) are modest, and many patients may have trouble tolerating cholinesterase inhibitors. Nevertheless, a trial of a cognitive enhancer should be considered in anyone with a diagnosis of dementia due to AD. A cognitive enhancer should also be considered for patients with PDD or DLB.

  - Cognitive enhancers are likely not effective in treating vascular dementia and MCI and should not be used in FTD.

  - Exercise may be the most effective psychosocial intervention for dementia. It should take place at least twice weekly and should include multiple activities, such as walking, stretching, and strength training. Cognitive stimulation in a group setting with an emphasis on social engagement may be helpful. Patients and their caregivers should consider switching to a Mediterranean diet.

- Except in the case of vitamin deficiency, there is no evidence to support supplementation with vitamins B_6, B_{12}, or folate. Vitamin E may improve functional outcomes but does not improve cognition in patients with dementia and does not slow progression from MCI to AD. Omega-3 fatty acid does not appear to be effective. There is insufficient evidence to support the use of ginkgo biloba, huperzine A, curcumin, or any other nutraceutical to address cognition in patients with dementia.
  - Because alcohol is neurotoxic, it should be avoided or consumed very sparingly.
- Functional impairment is universal in patients with dementia, and it worsens as the disease progresses. Patients' ADLs should be regularly assessed, and supports should be provided.
- Untreated pain may contribute to BPSD. Clinicians should screen patients with mild to moderate dementia for pain using a 0–10 numerical or similar rating scale. A structured tool such as the Pain Assessment in Advanced Dementia scale may be necessary for patients with severe dementia. Scheduling acetaminophen at dosages up to 3,000 mg/day may be effective at reducing pain and BPSD.
- Up to 62% of patients with dementia experience elder abuse, a potentially lethal condition. Clinicians should screen for elder abuse and, when suspected, notify appropriate local authorities for investigation.
- Patients should be encouraged to complete a health care POA, a financial POA, an advance directive, and a will. Clinicians can help patients discuss their wishes with their family members.
- BPSD affect 90% of patients with dementia and contribute to poor quality of life, caregiver burden, elder abuse, economic costs, and institutionalization.

RESOURCES FOR PATIENTS, FAMILIES, AND CAREGIVERS

Alosa Health: Elder Abuse and Dementia. Boston, MA, Alosa Health, 2017. Available at: https://alosahealth.org/clinical-modules/elder-abuse/. This well-written and visually appealing brochure informs older adults and their families regarding steps they can take to stay free of abuse and exploitation, red flags to watch for, and support that is available in case there is a concern. Alosa Health also instructs physicians in the academic detailing model of medical education, which involves content experts coming into clinical settings to educate practitioners.

Eldercare Locator (https://eldercare.acl.gov/Public/Index.aspx; 1-800-677-1116) is a list of local resources, compiled by the U.S. Administration on Aging, that can be searched by city and state or by zip code. The website also has brochures and fact sheets on a wide range of topics related to dementia care.

Mace N, Rabins P: The 36-Hour Day: A Family Guide to Caring for People Who Have Alzheimer Disease, Related Dementias, and Memory Loss, 6th Edition. Baltimore, MD, Johns Hopkins University Press, 2017. This gold-standard reference for caregivers includes education about what to expect in dementia and how to prepare for and respond to a range of situations. This book is quite long and could be overwhelming for an already very busy and tired caregiver. The next resource is an alternative that may be more approachable as a quick reference.

National Institute on Aging: Alzheimer's Disease and Related Dementias: Alzheimer's Caregiving. Bethesda, MD, National Institute on Aging, 2018. Available at: https://www.nia.nih.gov/health/alzheimers/caregiving. This web page is essentially a table of contents with links to pages covering more specific topics, such as legal and financial planning, driving safety, finding long-term care, self-care for caregivers, and many others.

National Institute on Aging: Home Safety Checklist for Alzheimer's Disease. Bethesda, MD, National Institute on Aging, 2017. Available at: https://www.nia.nih.gov/health/home-safety-checklist-alzheimers-disease. This web page provides a comprehensive list of steps to take within the home to help keep persons with AD and other dementias safe. It is organized as a room-by-room walkthrough of the home and the outside approaches to the home.

REFERENCES

2018 Physical Activity Guidelines Advisory Committee: 2018 Physical Activity Guidelines Advisory Committee Scientific Report. Rockville, MD, U.S. Office of Disease Prevention and Health Promotion, 2018

Alosa Health: Caring for Vulnerable Elders: Addressing Elder Abuse, Managing Dementia, Supporting Caregivers. Boston, MA, Alosa Health, 2017. Available at: http://alosahealth.org/uploads/Elder_Abuse_EvDoc_Final.pdf. Accessed March 24, 2018.

American Geriatrics Society Panel on Pharmacological Management of Persistent Pain in Older Persons: Pharmacological management of persistent pain in older persons. J Am Geriatr Soc 57(8):1331–1346, 2009 19573219

Baskys A, Cheng J-X: Pharmacological prevention and treatment of vascular dementia: approaches and perspectives. Exp Gerontol 47(11):887–891, 2012 22796225

Birks J, Grimley Evans J: Ginkgo biloba for cognitive impairment and dementia. Cochrane Database Syst Rev (1):CD003120, 2009 19160216

Buckley JS, Salpeter SR: A risk-benefit assessment of dementia medications: systematic review of the evidence. Drugs Aging 32(6):453–467, 2015 25941104

Burckhardt M, Herke M, Wustmann T, et al: Omega-3 fatty acids for the treatment of dementia. Cochrane Database Syst Rev 4(4):CD009002, 2016 27063583

Burton E, Cavalheri V, Adams R, et al: Effectiveness of exercise programs to reduce falls in older people with dementia living in the community: a systematic review and meta-analysis. Clin Interv Aging 10:421–434, 2015 25709416

Cummings JL, Morstorf T, Zhong K: Alzheimer's disease drug-development pipeline: few candidates, frequent failures. Alzheimers Res Ther 6(4):37, 2014 25024750

Dong X, Chen R, Simon MA: Elder abuse and dementia: a review of the research and health policy. Health Aff (Millwood) 33(4):642–649, 2014 24711326

Farina N, Llewellyn D, Isaac MG, et al: Vitamin E for Alzheimer's dementia and mild cognitive impairment. Cochrane Database Syst Rev (4):CD002854, 2017 28128435

Folstein MF, Folstein SE, McHugh PR: "Mini-mental state": a practical method for grading the cognitive state of patients for the clinician. J Psychiatr Res 12(3):189–198 1975 202204

Goodwill AM, Szoeke C: A systematic review and meta-analysis of the effect of low vitamin D on cognition. J Am Geriatr Soc 65(10):2161–2168, 2017 28758188

Hunt LJ, Covinsky KE, Yaffe K, et al: Pain in community-dwelling older adults with dementia: results from the National Health and Aging Trends Study. J Am Geriatr Soc 63(8):1503–1511, 2015 26200445

Husebo BS, Ballard C, Cohen-Mansfield J, et al: The response of agitated behavior to pain management in persons with dementia. Am J Geriatr Psychiatry 22(7):708–717, 2014 23611363

Kales HC, Gitlin LN, Lyketsos CG: Management of neuropsychiatric symptoms of dementia in clinical settings: recommendations from a multidisciplinary expert panel. J Am Geriatr Soc 62(4):762–769, 2014 24635665

Knopman DS: Donepezil 23 mg: an empty suit. Neurol Clin Pract 2(4):352–355, 2012 23634378

Löwe B, Kroenke K, Gräfe K: Detecting and monitoring depression with a two-item questionnaire (PHQ-2). J Psychosom Res 58(2):163–171 2005 15820844

Mace N, Rabins P: The 36-Hour Day: A Family Guide to Caring for People Who Have Alzheimer Disease, Related Dementias, and Memory Loss, 6th Edition. Baltimore, MD, Johns Hopkins University Press, 2017

McDermott O, Charlesworth G, Hogervorst E, et al: Psychosocial interventions for people with dementia: a synthesis of systematic reviews. Aging Ment Health 17:1–11, 2018 29338323

McGill Department of Family Medicine: Elder Abuse Suspicion Index (EASI). Montreal, Quebec, Canada, McGill University, 2018. Available at: https://www.mcgill.ca/familymed/research/projects/elder. Accessed August 4, 2018.

Morrin H, Fang T, Servant D, et al: Systematic review of the efficacy of non-pharmacological interventions in people with Lewy body dementia. Int Psychogeriatr 30(3):395–407, 2018 28988547

Morris JC: The Clinical Dementia Rating (CDR): current version and scoring rules. Neurology 43(11):2412–2414, 1993 8232972

Nardell M, Tampi RR: Pharmacological treatments for frontotemporal dementias: a systematic review of randomized controlled trials. Am J Alzheimers Dis Other Demen 29(2):123–132, 2014 24164931

National Institute for Health and Care Excellence: Dementia: Supporting People With Dementia and Their Carers in Health and Social Care. London, National Institute for Health and Care Excellence, 2006. Available at: https://www.nice.org.uk/guidance/cg42. Accessed March 18, 2018.

National Institute for Health and Care Excellence: Donepezil, Galantamine, Rivastigmine and Memantine for the Treatment of Alzheimer's Disease. London, National Institute for Health and Care Excellence, 2011. Available at: https://www.nice.org.uk/guidance/ta217. Accessed March 18, 2018.

Piazza-Gardner AK, Gaffud TJ, Barry AE: The impact of alcohol on Alzheimer's disease: a systematic review. Aging Ment Health 17(2):133–146, 2013 23171229

Qaseem A, Snow V, Cross JT Jr, et al: Current pharmacologic treatment of dementia: a clinical practice guideline from the American College of Physicians and the American Academy of Family Physicians. Ann Intern Med 148(5):370–378, 2008 18316755

Rabins PV, Blacker D, Rovner BW, et al: American Psychiatric Association practice guideline for the treatment of patients with Alzheimer's disease and other dementias, second edition. Am J Psychiatry 164 (12 suppl):5–56, 2007

Reisberg B: Functional assessment staging (FAST). Psychopharmacol Bull 24:653–659, 1988

Ridley NJ, Draper B, Withall A: Alcohol-related dementia: an update of the evidence. Alzheimers Res Ther 5(1):3, 2013 23347747

Sanders AE, Nininger J, Absher J, et al: Quality improvement in neurology: dementia management quality measurement set update. Am J Psychiatry 174(5):493–498, 2017 28457155

Sclan SG, Reisberg B: Functional Assessment Staging (FAST) in Alzheimer's disease: reliability, validity, and ordinality. Int Psychogeriatr 4 (suppl 1):55–69, 1992 1504288

Singh B, Parsaik AK, Mielke MM, et al: Association of Mediterranean diet with mild cognitive impairment and Alzheimer's disease: a systematic review and meta-analysis. J Alzheimers Dis 39(2):271–282, 2014 24164735

Tampi RR, Hassell C, Joshi P, et al: Analgesics in the management of behavioral and psychological symptoms of dementia: a perspective review. Drugs Context 6:212508, 2017 29209402

van de Rest O, Berendsen AA, Haveman-Nies A, et al: Dietary patterns, cognitive decline, and dementia: a systematic review. Adv Nutr 6(2):154–168, 2015 25770254

Wang H-F, Yu J-T, Tang S-W, et al: Efficacy and safety of cholinesterase inhibitors and memantine in cognitive impairment in Parkinson's disease, Parkinson's disease dementia, and dementia with Lewy bodies: systematic review with meta-analysis and trial sequential analysis. J Neurol Neurosurg Psychiatry 86(2):135–143, 2015 24828899

Warden V, Hurley AC, Volicer L: Development and psychometric evaluation of the Pain Assessment in Advanced Dementia (PAINAD) scale. J Am Med Dir Assoc 4(1):9–15, 2003 12807591

Ware LJ, Herr KA, Booker SS, et al: Psychometric evaluation of the Revised Iowa Pain Thermometer (IPT-R) in a sample of diverse cognitively intact and impaired older adults: a pilot study. Pain Manag Nurs 16(4):475–482, 2015 26256217

Woods B, O'Philbin L, Farrell EM, et al: Reminiscence therapy for dementia. Cochrane Database Syst Rev 3:CD001120, 2018 29493789

Yaffe MJ, Wolfson C, Lithwick M, et al: Development and validation of a tool to improve physician identification of elder abuse: the Elder Abuse Suspicion Index (EASI). J Elder Abuse Negl 20(3):276–300, 2008 18928055

Young JJ, Lavakumar M, Tampi D, et al: Frontotemporal dementia: latest evidence and clinical implications. Ther Adv Psychopharmacol 8(1):33–48, 2018 29344342

Zhang DM, Ye JX, Mu JS, et al: Efficacy of vitamin B supplementation on cognition in elderly patients with cognitive-related diseases. J Geriatr Psychiatry Neurol 30(1):50–59, 2017 28248558

CHAPTER 3

INTRODUCTION TO BEHAVIORAL AND PSYCHOLOGICAL SYMPTOMS OF DEMENTIA

Précis

Behavioral and psychological symptoms are common in dementia, worsen the quality of life of patients and their caregivers, decrease the ability of patients to care for themselves, can pose a significant hazard to safety, and may increase the risk of death. The most common behavioral and psychological symptoms of dementia (BPSD) include apathy, depression, delusions, and agitation; other important symptoms include verbal and physical aggression, hallucinations, anxiety, irritability, disinhibition, restlessness, wandering, sleep disturbances, changes in eating, and refusal of care or medications. The prevalence of BPSD peaks during the moderate stage of dementia, but symptoms can be present during any stage and can also wax and wane over time. Understanding how BPSD arise is essential for ultimately developing a plan to address and even prevent BPSD, and there are a number of models to aid in this process.

BACKGROUND AND TERMINOLOGY

Although *dementia* is defined as the combination of cognitive impairment and functional impairment, a strong case can be made that behavior changes and psychological manifestations are prevalent enough to consider them intrinsic to dementia. Approximately 90% of patients with Alzheimer's disease (AD) experience clinically significant BPSD between diagnosis and death (Kales et al. 2014). DSM-5 criteria for the diagnosis of major neurocognitive disorder (American Psychiatric Association 2013) match what is described in this book as dementia and rest on the presence of one or more domains of cognitive impairment leading to functional impairment. However, it is noteworthy that early criteria recognized the prominence of BPSD: for example, the 1984 National Institute of Neurological and Communicative Disorders and Stroke–Alzheimer's Disease and Related Disorders Association criteria for the diagnosis of AD listed the following clinical features as consistent with probable AD: depression; insomnia; delusions; hallucinations; catastrophic verbal, emotional, or physical outbursts; sexual disorders; and weight loss (McKhann et al. 1984). In two of the most common other causes of dementia—dementia with Lewy bodies (DLB) and frontotemporal dementia (FTD)—such symptoms *are* part of the current diagnostic criteria (see the section "Making the Diagnosis" in Chapter 1).

In this book, I use the term *behavioral and psychological symptoms of dementia*, but many writers refer to these as *neuropsychiatric symptoms* of dementia. Although the term *agitation* is often used broadly to refer to BPSD, this term refers only to a subset of relevant BPSD and misses important symptoms such as depression, anxiety, sleep-wake disturbance, and so on. The Neuropsychiatric Inventory (NPI), a rating scale commonly used in research studies of BPSD, categorizes the symptoms as follows (Kaufer et al. 2000):

- Aberrant motor behaviors
- Agitation or aggression
- Anxiety
- Apathy
- Appetite disorder
- Delusions
- Depression
- Disinhibition
- Elation/euphoria
- Hallucinations
- Irritability
- Sleep disorder

Agitation or aggression can be verbal (e.g., yelling, swearing, making inappropriate comments) or physical (e.g., pacing, throwing objects, grabbing, hitting, biting). Other concerning or problematic behaviors include wandering, refusing medications, refusing assistance with activities of daily living (ADLs), and pathological laughing and crying (PLC). *Sundowning* refers to behaviors that arise in the late afternoon or early evening (e.g., restlessness, confusion, verbal aggression, physical aggression). Obtaining a clear history of these symptoms from patients and caregivers is critical to understanding the cause of the symptoms and the best ways to address them; I recommend rich descriptions of these behaviors coupled with an understanding of the broader categories of behaviors. I discuss this topic further in the section "Specifying and Characterizing BPSD" in Chapter 4.

EPIDEMIOLOGY OF BPSD

In general, the prevalence of BPSD increases over the course of illness, peaking in moderate dementia (Figure 3–1; Okura et al. 2010). The distribution of specific BPSD varies by stage: depression is the most common symptom in mild cognitive impairment (MCI) and in mild dementia; delusions are the most common symptoms in moderate dementia; and apathy and agitation are the most common symptoms in severe dementia. As shown in Table 3–1, the most common symptoms overall are apathy (estimated prevalence of 49% in patients with AD), depression (42%), and aggression (40%) (Zhao et al. 2016). The sum of the prevalence estimates for all the symptoms listed in Table 3–1 is much higher than 100%, which indicates that multiple symptoms can be present at the same time; in fact, some clustering of symptoms (e.g., depression, anxiety, and insomnia) can take place. Symptoms may wax and wane over time in a somewhat unpredictable fashion. I discuss each of the BPSD in greater detail in the section "Presentation of Specific BPSD," later in this chapter.

Much of what is known about BPSD comes from studying patients with AD. It appears that the overall prevalence rates of BPSD are similar in vascular dementia, though depression and apathy may be more common in vascular dementia than in AD, perhaps due to cerebrovascular disease disrupting functional networks involved in emotion regulation and the initiation/execution of activities (Tiel et al. 2015). FTD is notable for behavioral disturbance, with higher rates of disinhibition, aberrant motor behavior, and eating disturbances than in AD (Bang et al. 2015). Hallucinations are far more common in Lewy body disease (LBD) than in other causes of dementia and are part of the diagnostic criteria for DLB; sleep disturbance due to rapid eye movement (REM) sleep behavior disorder is also common (McKeith et al. 2017).

EFFECTS OF BPSD ON PATIENTS, CAREGIVERS, AND SOCIETY

Unquestionably, patients themselves suffer the greatest toll from BPSD. Consequences of BPSD include emotional distress, diminished quality of

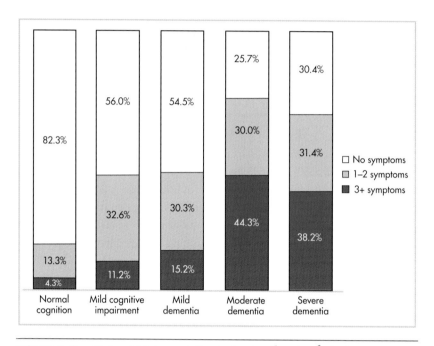

FIGURE 3–1. Natural history of the behavioral and psychological symptoms of dementia (BPSD): prevalence by cognitive status.

The prevalence of clinically significant BPSD varies by cognitive status. The categories include subjects with no BPSD, one or two BPSD, and three or more BPSD in the past month. The Neuropsychiatric Inventory was used to determine the frequency, severity, and caregiver distress associated with each symptom. A symptom was defined as "clinically significant" when the product of the frequency score (4-point scale) and the severity score (3-point scale) was greater than or equal to 4.

Source.   Adapted from Okura et al. 2010.

life, accidental injury, more rapid progression of cognitive impairment, greater functional impairment (contributing to higher risk of institutionalization), more frequent hospitalizations, higher risk of abuse and neglect (including self-neglect), and decreased survival (Kales et al. 2014). The economic burden is staggering, with BPSD accounting for 30% of the cost of care of people with dementia in the community.

BPSD also pose a significant burden to caregivers (Cheng 2017). Being a caregiver for someone with dementia is stressful in and of itself; for example, 34% of caregivers for patients with AD have depression and 44% have anxiety (Sallim et al. 2015). The presence of behavioral problems in patients only increases stress further. BPSD may be more disturbing to caregivers than cognitive and functional impairments of care recipients, at least

TABLE 3–1. Prevalence of specific behavioral and psychological symptoms of dementia (BPSD)

Symptom	Percentage
Apathy	49
Depression	42
Aggression	40
Sleep disorder	39
Anxiety	39
Irritability	36
Appetite disorder	34
Aberrant motor behavior	32
Delusions	31
Disinhibition	17
Hallucinations	16
Euphoria	7

Note. Estimates of prevalence are pooled from 48 studies of BPSD in Alzheimer's disease, using the Neuropsychiatric Inventory.
Source. Data from Zhao et al. 2016.

in the early to middle stages of dementia. By later stages of dementia, greater functional impairments (and the associated increase in time spent caregiving) may be the greater driver of caregiver burden. BPSD and functional impairments may also interact with each other: assisting someone with ADLs is more challenging when that person also has BPSD. Although the literature is not conclusive on this point, clinical experience indicates that caregivers may find specific BPSD to be particularly distressing, including the following: aggression, delusions (especially paranoid ideation and delusions of infidelity), irritability, depression, and apathy. Sleep disturbances can be particularly troublesome for caregivers, because their own sleep is thereby interrupted. All these factors contribute to increasing the risk of abuse or neglect by caregivers and to decreasing the time to institutionalization of patients. Finally, caregivers experience economic consequences, such as decreased income from employment (Kales et al. 2014). Clearly, BPSD can take a toll on caregivers and can have profound impacts on patient-caregiver relationships.

ETIOLOGICAL MODELS OF BPSD

Behavioral and psychological symptoms arise from the interplay among the neurobiological alterations of dementia, premorbid personality traits, increased stressors and diminished capacity to adaptively respond to them, altered interpersonal relationships and supports, unmet needs, and co-occurring medical problems. Although the exact details vary among specific BPSD (see the next section, "Presentation of Specific BPSD"), it is possible to make some generalizations about how BPSD arise.

The *behavioral model* posits that behaviors arise in response to or following specific antecedents and that the behaviors in turn lead to or are followed by consequences (Figure 3–2) (Teri et al. 1998). This can serve as a simple yet powerful explanatory model to patients, family members, and other caregivers. A clinician can use this model to elicit symptoms from caregivers and to better understand the contexts in which symptoms arise and how people respond to the symptoms (see Chapter 4 for a detailed discussion of this approach). For example, a caregiver may express concern that the person with dementia has become physically aggressive, specifically pushing the caregiver away (behavior). The behavior occurs each morning, when the caregiver attempts to help the person with dementia choose clothes to wear and then put on the clothes (antecedents). The person with dementia refuses to put on clothes for the day, walking around the house in pajamas all day, leading to frustration and embarrassment for the caregiver (consequences). This model leads to a therapeutic approach that involves carefully observing target behaviors, identifying strategies to reduce behaviors, and implementing these strategies (Teri et al. 1998).

A more complex approach, which has been found to be helpful in training caregivers how to analyze and respond to BPSD, is the *progressively lowered stress threshold model* (Smith et al. 2004). This model posits that behaviors arise from a mismatch between the stressors of the environment and the capacity of a person with dementia to appropriately respond to those stressors (Figure 3–3). A person with dementia exhibits three types of behaviors: *baseline behaviors* (presumably not problematic), *anxious behaviors* (as the person approaches his or her stress threshold), and *dysfunctional behaviors* (once beyond the stress threshold). Dysfunctional behaviors may include repetitive behaviors, agitation, combativeness, situationally inappropriate behaviors, "catastrophic reactions" (see the section "Anxiety and Irritability" later in this chapter), and sleep disturbances. Because of cognitive impairments (e.g., being unable to recognize objects and how to use them, being unable to recognize those who ought to be familiar) and exec-

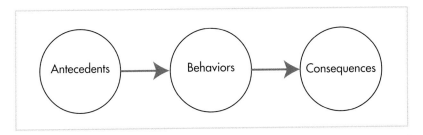

FIGURE 3–2. How behavioral and psychological symptoms of dementia arise: behavioral model.

A simple behavioral model posits that *behaviors* arise after or in response to *antecedents* and that *consequences* arise after or in response to *behaviors*. Positive and negative reinforcers (not pictured) lead to increased and decreased frequency of behavior, respectively.

utive dysfunction (e.g., decreased ability to select an appropriate behavior for the circumstances), the threshold at which stress leads to dysfunctional behavior is progressively lowered over the course of dementia. Similarly, the stress threshold may decrease over the course of each day, which may help explain why dysfunctional behaviors can be worse in the late afternoon or early evening (i.e., sundowning—see the section "Disturbances of Sleep-Wake Cycle" later in this chapter). Stressors may include fatigue, changes in routine or in the environment, changes in caregivers, excess stimulation, medical problems, medication side effects, and depression and/or anxiety in response to loss. This model has led to recommendations for caregivers with respect to identifying and modifying stressors, monitoring for increasing anxiety and agitation among persons with dementia, and promoting adaptive responses for both persons with dementia and their caregivers (see the section "Support and Education of Family and Other Caregivers" in Chapter 5 for further discussion).

The *unmet needs model* argues that BPSD result when a person with dementia has an unmet need that cannot be expressed in a typical way; the caregiver in turn has difficulty recognizing that there is an unmet need driving the behavior (Kovach et al. 2005). Background (predisposing) factors include memory problems, language impairment, premorbid personality traits, and comorbid medical problems (Figure 3–4). Proximal (precipitating) factors in the current environment and situation could include pain, fatigue, infection, dehydration, overstimulation, changes in caregivers, and so on. Together, these factors turn *primary needs* into *need-driven, dementia-compromised behaviors*—that is, BPSD. The model further argues that when primary needs go unmet, they develop into *secondary needs* with their own

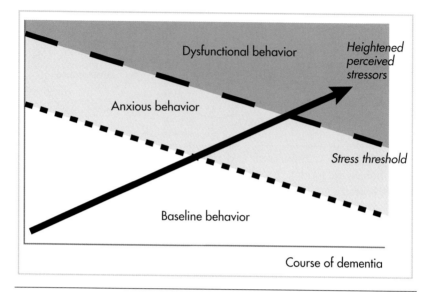

FIGURE 3–3.   How behavioral and psychological symptoms of dementia arise: progressively lowered stress threshold model.

Over the course of dementia, the threshold for stress progressively diminishes. As the perceived level of stress approaches the stress threshold, anxious behaviors become more frequent. Once the perceived level of stress crosses the stress threshold, dysfunctional behaviors such as agitation arise.

Source.   Adapted from Smith M, Gerdner LA, Hall GR, Buckwalter KC: "History, Development, and Future of the Progressively Lowered Stress Threshold: A Conceptual Model for Dementia Care." *Journal of the American Geriatrics Society* 52(10):1755–1760, 2004. © The American Geriatrics Society. Used with permission.

associated dementia-compromised behaviors. For example, a person with dementia who is thirsty and has trouble appropriately expressing a need for fluids (primary need) may manifest repetitive (seemingly purposeless) movements (primary need-driven, dementia-compromised behavior). Eventually, the person may develop constipation and abdominal pain that require a stool softener (secondary need) and that manifest as physical aggression (secondary need-driven, dementia-compromised behavior). Another risk of not recognizing an unmet need is that caregivers may respond in an ineffective or even counterproductive way; in the example cited, perhaps the caregiver seeks a prescription for antipsychotic medication to treat the physical aggression, which not only does not address the underlying issues of thirst and constipation but also could exacerbate matters by resulting in side effects of dry mouth and constipation. As I discuss in the section "Support and Education of Family and Other Caregivers" in Chapter 5, the

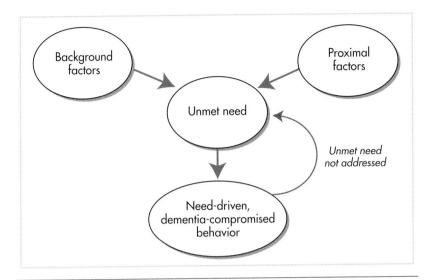

FIGURE 3–4. How behavioral and psychological symptoms of dementia (BPSD) arise: unmet needs model.

The unmet needs model argues that the BPSD (here referred to as need-driven, dementia-compromised behaviors) represent signals of underlying, unmet needs. The unmet needs arise from predisposing/background factors (e.g., cognitive impairment) and precipitating/proximal factors (e.g., pain). When unmet needs are not identified and addressed, BPSD may create new unmet needs, leading to a cascade of unmet needs and behavioral problems.
Source. Adapted from Kovach et al. 2005.

resulting clinical approach includes educating caregivers about the warning signs of unmet needs and developing a treatment plan to address these needs.

The *Wisconsin Star Method*, an expansion of the construct of biopsychosocial formulation used in psychiatric diagnosis, argues that BPSD (and other geriatric syndromes, such as frequent falls) arise as a result of the interactions among 1) medical factors, 2) medications (both therapeutic effects and side effects), 3) psychological factors (including premorbid personality structure), 4) social factors (e.g., interpersonal or environmental stressors), and 5) behavioral or psychiatric symptoms (Howell 2015). The five sets of factors (both risk and protective) are arrayed around the star to demonstrate their interrelationships—and to identify targets for interventions (Figure 3–5). Medical factors include vision and hearing loss, acute and chronic pain, malnutrition, dehydration, urinary retention, urinary incontinence, and constipation. Medications such as opioids, sedative-hypnotics, and medications with anticholinergic effects can cause or exacerbate BPSD,

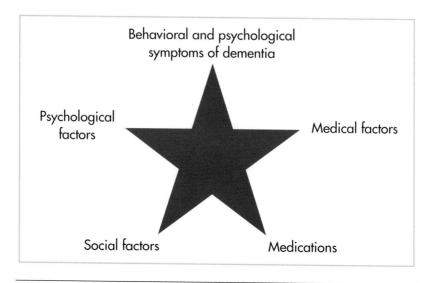

FIGURE 3–5. How behavioral and psychological symptoms of dementia (BPSD) arise: Wisconsin Star Method.

The Wisconsin Star Method highlights the interrelationships among psychological factors, social factors, medical factors, and medications in the genesis of BPSD. These may be protective factors or risk factors. The Madison Veterans Administration Hospital, the University of Wisconsin School of Medicine and Public Health, the Division of Mental Health and Substance Abuse Services of the Wisconsin Department of Health Services, National Alliance on Mental Illness (NAMI) Wisconsin, and members of the Wisconsin Geriatric Psychiatry Initiative have provided in-kind support for the development of the Wisconsin Star Method.

whereas medications such as antidepressants, cognitive enhancers, or antipsychotics might reduce frequency and intensity of BPSD. Psychological factors include loneliness, grief, boredom, fear, and premorbid personality traits. Finally, social factors include interactions with family members and other caregivers (both positive and negative), changes in the environment or routine, and so on. The Wisconsin Star Method can serve as a powerful educational and clinical tool for health care providers attempting to understand and address BPSD.

Results from studies of the neurobiological correlates of BPSD, including neuroanatomic abnormalities, neurochemical alterations, and genetic risk factors, are not completely consistent. Furthermore, neurobiological abnormalities appear to vary by type of BPSD (and by the cause of dementia). I briefly summarize the literature here (Boublay et al. 2016; Casanova et al. 2011; Rosenberg et al. 2015):

1. *Agitation:* It appears that atrophy of the frontal cortex, insula, cingulate cortex, amygdala, and hippocampus is associated with agitation—implicating networks involved in emotion regulation, assessing salience of threats, and problem solving. Decreased cholinergic activity, decreased serotonergic activity, and increased tau protein have also been associated with agitation. These changes appear to parallel the core pathology of AD itself.

2. *Apathy:* Damage to the anterior cingulate cortex (as evidenced by amyloid burden, hypoperfusion, decreased white matter integrity, and atrophy) has been consistently found in studies of apathy. Other regions implicated include the frontal lobes in general and the orbitofrontal cortex in particular. Other associations with apathy include decreased dopaminergic activity in the putamen, increased tau protein in cerebrospinal fluid, and the presence of vascular risk factors.

3. *Delusions:* Findings are similar to those for agitation, with abnormalities in the frontal cortex and anterior cingulate cortex, plus disturbances in dopamine signaling and neuronal loss in the hippocampus and the parahippocampal gyrus.

4. *Depression:* Atrophy of the hippocampus and of the anterior cingulate cortex has been associated with depression. Vascular disease in the white matter and vascular risk factors have also been associated with depression.

The *APOE** ε4 allele has been associated with AD; its relationship with BPSD in general and specific BPSD is less clear, with contradictory findings from a number of studies (Panza et al. 2012). With respect to premorbid personality traits, the most consistent finding is that neuroticism (proneness to emotional arousal and negativity) is associated with disturbances in mood and with aggression (Osborne et al. 2010). As noted earlier in this section, medical conditions may contribute to BPSD, including pain, dehydration, constipation, vision loss, hearing loss, and infections.

Interestingly, caregivers attribute BPSD to a wide variety of factors, including neurobiological causes (e.g., "wiring problems in the brain"), comorbid medical problems (e.g., hearing or vision loss), psychological reaction to dementia (e.g., uncertainty, frustration, loss of independence), shifting or losing social roles and relationships, and environmental changes—and they may believe behaviors to be volitional (Polenick et al. 2018). Cultural backgrounds of caregivers may also influence caregivers' explanations of behavior (Suzuki et al. 2015). Exploring caregivers' understanding of BPSD and educating them about the causes of BPSD are critical components of addressing BPSD.

PRESENTATION OF SPECIFIC BPSD

Dementia disrupts emotions and affects behaviors in many ways. Clustering BPSD into categories such as affective disturbance, psychosis, and agitation may be useful (e.g., in treatment planning), but BPSD may be best thought of as protean manifestations of a fundamental, underlying disruption in the ability to regulate emotion and behavior. BPSD wax and wane over time, and the specific symptoms may also change with progression of dementia (which may account for the high placebo response rate found in drug trials of BPSD—more on this in Chapter 5). For example, a patient with prominent dysphoria and anxiety may later become paranoid, which may initially manifest as withdrawal and later as screaming and punching, and so on. The following subsections present a comprehensive list of BPSD, and Table 3–2 summarizes these symptoms.

Depression

Feeling sad, hopeless, or discouraged is not uncommon among people with dementia, especially in early stages of dementia, when the person may be aware of changes in memory and functioning. Depression may be a psychological reaction to loss: loss of memory, loss of ability to care for oneself, loss of independence, and loss of loved ones. The hippocampus, which degenerates over the course of AD, not only is responsible for encoding memories but also is part of the limbic circuitry involved in emotion regulation. As noted, cerebrovascular disease may disrupt white matter tracts linking prefrontal cortex with subcortical structures, thereby also affecting emotion regulation. Depression in AD presents similarly to a major depressive episode, with symptoms including low mood, changes in appetite, changes in sleep, psychomotor restlessness or slowing, fatigue, worthlessness, hopelessness, guilt, and suicidal ideation. Unlike major depressive episode, depression in AD may also include irritability. Criteria for the depression in AD have been developed; they include, in addition to the features just listed, decreased positive affect or pleasure in response to social contacts and activities (similar to anhedonia in major depressive episode) and social isolation or withdrawal (Olin et al. 2002).

The incidence of suicidal ideation increases slightly soon after the diagnosis of dementia, but the risk of suicide gradually decreases as the disease progresses, likely due to executive dysfunction interfering with the ability to carry out a plan to end one's life (Seyfried et al. 2011). Nevertheless, patients with dementia and depression should be screened for suicidal ide-

TABLE 3–2. Overview of specific behavioral and psychological symptoms of dementia

Symptom	Presentation	Comments
Depression	Similar to DSM-5 criteria for major depressive disorder, except that irritability may also be present; suicide risk highest immediately after diagnosis of dementia, decreases as dementia progresses	Self-report measures (PHQ–9, GDS) become increasingly unreliable as dementia progresses. Consider using CSDD instead.
Apathy	Loss of motivation and interest; less interest in others; less likely to initiate and engage in conversation; less affectionate or emotional	Psychological hallmarks of depression (hopelessness, worthlessness, guilt) are usually not present. Family may be more upset than patient.
Verbal aggression and other vocalizations	Screaming, swearing, making repetitive statements, moaning, laughing inappropriately	Consider pathological laughing and crying (listed later in table) as an alternate explanation.
Physical aggression, agitation, and other aberrant motor behaviors	Wide range of behaviors, including intruding upon others, slamming doors, throwing objects, kicking, pushing, scratching, biting, wandering, fidgeting, restlessness, pacing, refusing medications, refusing help with ADLs, sexually inappropriate behavior	Assess risk of harm to self and others. Some caregivers may incorrectly refer to repetitive behaviors as obsessive-compulsive.

TABLE 3–2. Overview of specific behavioral and psychological symptoms of dementia *(continued)*

Symptom	Presentation	Comments
Disturbances of sleep-wake cycle	Sleeping during the day, up at night (Alzheimer's disease); agitation at night (REM sleep behavior disorder; seen in LBD)	Sundowning involves increasing confusion and behavioral symptoms in the late afternoon or early evening, perhaps due to circadian disturbance or to decreased stress threshold over the course of the day.
Anxiety and irritability	Worry that is difficult to control, repetitive statements or questions, being fearful when alone, following loved ones around the house, becoming upset when a loved one leaves the house or even the room the patient is in, fearing that one is going to be abandoned, avoiding anxiety-provoking situations, panic attacks, frequent complaining, arguing with others, sudden flashes of anger, getting upset easily	Catastrophic reaction is severe emotional outburst and associated physical agitation that seem inappropriate or out of proportion to the triggering event.
Delusions and hallucinations	Delusions include paranoia, infidelity, believing one's home is not one's own, and misidentification syndromes; visual hallucinations more common than auditory hallucinations	Hallucinations are more prominent in DLB.
Elation, euphoria, and disinhibition	Excessively good mood, telling jokes inappropriately, overly familiar with others, socially inappropriate behavior	Consider possibility of FTD, frontal lobe stroke, TBI, or bipolar disorder.

TABLE 3–2. Overview of specific behavioral and psychological symptoms of dementia *(continued)*

Symptom	Presentation	Comments
Pathological laughing and crying	Sudden and spontaneous crying or (less commonly) laughing, without associated emotional experience of sadness or joy	Also known as pseudobulbar palsy, pseudobulbar affect, or emotional incontinence, this behavior may arise in FTD, TBI, ALS, or MS.
Alterations in appetite and eating	Decreased olfaction and appetite, decreased ability to prepare meals, weight loss, dysphagia; in FTD, overeating, carbohydrate craving, or eating only very specific foods can occur	Consider side effects of acetylcholinesterase inhibitors (nausea, stomach upset, weight loss).

Note. ADLs=activities of daily living; ALS=amyotrophic lateral sclerosis; CSDD=Cornell Scale for Depression in Dementia; DLB=dementia with Lewy bodies; FTD=frontotemporal dementia; GDS=Geriatric Depression Scale; LBD=Lewy body disease; MS=multiple sclerosis; PHQ–9=Patient Health Questionnaire–9; REM=rapid eye movement; TBI=traumatic brain injury.

ation, which in turn should be appropriately addressed (see the section "Interventions by Symptom" in Chapter 5).

The mental status examination of a patient with dementia and depression may include tearfulness, downcast gaze, psychomotor slowing, furrowed brow, and a report of low mood. The Cornell Scale for Depression in Dementia (Alexopoulos et al. 1988) may be used to identify and measure the severity of depression. Other instruments, such as the Patient Health Questionnaire–9 (Spitzer et al. 1999) and the Geriatric Depression Scale (Sheikh and Yesavage 1986), may not have adequate sensitivity for depression in patients with moderate to severe dementia.

Apathy

Apathy is best understood as a marked loss of motivation. It is characterized by a patient initiating fewer activities and having overall less goal-directed behavior. Patients with apathy are less interested in their usual activities (and therefore apathy may overlap with *anhedonia*, which is the loss of pleasure from activities that is found in depression); less interested in the activities and plans of others, including family members and friends; less likely to initiate and engage in conversation; and less affectionate or emotional.

Distinguishing among apathy, depression, and the typical cognitive changes of dementia can be challenging, though the following observations may be helpful: Guilt, worthlessness, and hopelessness—the psychological hallmarks of depression—are typically not present in patients with apathy or dementia alone. Memory loss can interfere with one's ability to participate in activities and to engage with others, but patients without apathy will typically voice frustration with or concern about these problems. I have found that one of the hallmarks of apathy is that patients may not be particularly distressed about their apathy (i.e., they are apathetic about being apathetic), whereas their family members are frustrated and even infuriated by their loved ones' apathy and lack of concern about it.

Verbal Aggression and Other Vocalizations

A patient with dementia may scream or swear at others—or at no one in particular. Comments may be sarcastic, derogatory, insulting, insensitive, or sexually inappropriate. In patients with hallucinations or paranoia, vocalizations may represent attempts to communicate with what they perceive to be other people.

Repetitive statements, complaints, and questions may be due to forgetting that one has just said the same thing or asked the same question, or may represent anxiety or even paranoia; such statements and questions can be especially frustrating to caregivers. Moaning may indicate that the patient is in pain and otherwise unable to express it. Laughing inappropriately can lead to embarrassment for the patient and bewilderment or even anger for others; PLC, described later, should also be considered.

Physical Aggression, Agitation, and Other Aberrant Motor Behaviors

Of all the BPSD, nothing raises alarm as much as physical aggression does—and rightfully so, because patients and those around may be at risk of serious injury. Such behavior is usually a marker of severe distress in patients. It frightens caregivers and, in institutional settings, other residents. Behaviors may have antecedents/precipitants (e.g., perceived threats to privacy or self-determination, such as when a caregiver attempts to assist a patient with personal care or to set a limit on other behaviors) or may arise spontaneously (and sometimes even quite suddenly). Specific behaviors include entering others' rooms inappropriately, intruding on the care of others, slamming doors, taking items from others, throwing objects, kicking furniture or others, pushing others, scratching others, and biting others. Aggressive patients may accidentally harm themselves, especially if they are older, frail, osteoporotic, or unsteady on their feet. They may also injure family members, professional caregivers, and other residents. Such behaviors may lead to emergency medical services being activated, emergency department visits, hospitalizations, and even the involvement of law enforcement.

A consensus definition for *agitation* includes 1) meeting criteria for dementia or MCI; 2) excess motor activity, verbal aggression, or physical aggression associated with emotional distress and present for at least 2 weeks; 3) severity great enough to produce disability beyond that due to cognitive impairment; and 4) not being solely due to another psychiatric disorder, "suboptimal care conditions," medical condition, or physiological effects of a substance (Cummings et al. 2015).

Wandering—leaving one's residence without needed supervision—affects up to 62% of patients with dementia and can be quite dangerous to patients and alarming to caregivers (Borsje et al. 2015). Patients may wander because they are bored, they are searching for someone (e.g., a family member, including one who has passed away), they hope to return to a prior home, they are following a routine (e.g., walking to the grocery store), or they are anxious (e.g., fearful that someone is breaking into the home). Wandering can occur at night when caregivers are asleep or during dangerous weather conditions such as frigid weather, snowstorms, severe thunderstorms, and excessive heat or humidity. Patients may not leave the residence dressed properly for the conditions and therefore may be at risk of exposure even when the weather is not inherently dangerous. Other hazards include falling and being struck by a vehicle. Patients who are still driving pose additional risks, as discussed in the section "Assessing and Supporting Activities of Daily Living" in Chapter 2 and the section "Driving Safety" in Chapter 6.

Other motor behaviors may be less immediately concerning but can be precursors to the behaviors just described: fidgeting, restlessness, repetitive purposeless behaviors, pacing, refusing medications, refusing help with ADLs, being otherwise uncooperative or resistant, hoarding or hiding objects, calling emergency medical services or family members to seek help, and inappropriate sexual behaviors (including public masturbation or exposing oneself, lewd or suggestive gestures or comments, and sexually touching or grabbing others).

Note that caregivers sometimes refer to repetitive speech and behaviors as obsessive or compulsive; however, these symptoms are not consistent with true obsessive-compulsive disorder. Patients with dementia rarely describe experiencing anxiety caused by intrusive thoughts (obsessions) that is temporarily relieved by compensatory behaviors (compulsions). In the terminology of Parkinson disease, *punding* refers to purposeless, repetitive behaviors found more commonly in patients treated with levodopa than in those not treated with levodopa, suggesting dopaminergic dysfunction as a cause.

Disturbances of Sleep-Wake Cycle

Alterations in the sleep-wake cycle are common in dementia. AD is associated with degeneration of the suprachiasmatic nucleus, a part of the hypothalamus responsible for the circadian rhythm. Fragmentation of the sleep-wake cycle, including sleeping during the day and being up at night, can occur early in the course of AD and may become progressively worse. LBD is associated with REM sleep behavior disorder, wherein patients may shout, wander, and become physically aggressive at night. Being up at night also leads to increased risk of falls and to the possibility of wandering out of the residence. Problems with sleep take a significant toll on caregivers, who might otherwise have found respite in being able to get a good night's rest. Sundowning (sometimes referred to as sundowner's syndrome) may also be considered a disturbance of circadian rhythms, with symptoms of confusion and agitation arising in the late afternoon or early evening. Delirium may also interfere with the sleep-wake cycle, with fluctuations in arousal, excessive sleep during the daytime, and hyperarousal at night.

Anxiety and Irritability

Anxiety disorders are among the most common mental disorders in the general population. Dementia is an incredibly stressful condition, so the high prevalence of anxiety among patients with dementia is not surprising. Anxiety may manifest as worry that is difficult to control, repetitive statements or questions, being fearful when alone, following loved ones around the house, becoming upset when a loved one leaves the house or even the room the patient is in, fearing that one is going to be abandoned, avoiding anxiety-provoking situations (e.g., leaving the house or, in the case of fear of falling, even walking), and panic attacks. Caregivers' attempts to console or reassure patients may fail because amnesia leads to forgetting the consolation or reassurance but not the underlying source of anxiety. For patients who retain awareness of their cognitive impairments, the prospect of further cognitive decline can provoke anxiety (in particular if they have witnessed others who have dementia). As noted, true obsessions and compulsions are rare in dementia.

One of the cognitive changes in dementia, in particular when the frontal lobes are affected, is diminished ability to tolerate frustration—which may manifest as irritability. Signs of irritability include frequent complaining, arguing with others, sudden flashes of anger, and getting upset easily. The term *catastrophic reaction* refers to severe emotional outbursts and associated physical agitation that seem inappropriate or out of proportion to the triggering event. Irritability may also be found in depression and anxiety—in other words, there can be substantial overlap among these emotional experiences.

Delusions and Hallucinations

In younger patients, delusions and hallucinations are the hallmarks of psychotic disorders such as schizophrenia, psychotic depression, mania with psychotic features, and substance-induced psychotic disorders. Onset of these disorders in late life is relatively uncommon, so the presence of psychosis in an older adult should immediately raise the possibility of dementia (or delirium).

The most common delusions in dementia are delusions of theft (when in fact the patient has misplaced the object thought to have been stolen), delusions of infidelity (namely, the belief that one's spouse or partner is having an affair) or jealousy, persecutory delusions, and misidentification delusions (e.g., home is not one's own, stranger living in the home, imposter has replaced a family member or friend, deceased relatives or friends are still alive). One curious aspect of most of these delusions is the role of amnesia: a patient who forgets where he has put his wallet accuses his wife of intentionally stealing; a patient who no longer recognizes her husband believes that there is a stranger in her bed; a patient who forgets that he has already received a medication accuses his caregiver of not giving him the medication; and so on. The involvement of memory loss has led such delusions to be referred to as "paramnestic."

Diagnostic criteria for the psychosis of AD have been developed (though not included in DSM-5): 1) presence of auditory/visual hallucinations and/or delusions; 2) meeting criteria for dementia due to AD; 3) hallucinations/delusions have not been present continuously since before the onset of dementia; 4) hallucinations/delusions have been present for at least 1 month; 5) not meeting criteria for schizophrenia, schizoaffective disorder, delusional disorder, or mood disorder with psychotic features; 6) not occurring exclusively during delirium; and 7) not better accounted for by another medical condition or the direct physiological effects of a substance (Jeste and Finkel 2000).

A clinician may find it difficult to determine if an accusation made against a caregiver is factual or delusional. For example, a patient who insists that a caregiver is trying to harm him or her may be paranoid or may be quite right. A social services (or even police) investigation may be required to determine the truth. Delusions may be associated with depression, anxiety, irritability, verbal aggression, physical aggression, and wandering.

Delusions less commonly seen in dementia include grandiose delusions, erotomanic delusions, religious delusions, and somatic delusions (e.g., the belief that one is rotting on the inside). The presence of one of these should raise the possibility that the patient has a primary psychiatric disorder such as psychotic depression, bipolar disorder, or schizophrenia. Some patients with Parkinson disease report "presence delusions"—that is, the sense that someone else is in the room, without associated auditory or visual hallucinations.

Hallucinations are a hallmark of DLB but may also occur in other causes of dementia. Visual hallucinations are more common than auditory hallucinations; olfactory, tactile, and gustatory hallucinations are rare. In the case of DLB, visual hallucinations are often very vivid and detailed and sometimes quite frightening. Visual hallucinations may be of animals, children, or other people. Auditory hallucinations are typically voices of others, though musical hallucinations have been reported following stroke. The presence of hallucinations should also raise the possibility of delirium, medication side effects, and Charles Bonnet syndrome (visual hallucinations due to vision loss).

Elation, Euphoria, and Disinhibition

Elation and *euphoria* refer to excessively good mood and feeling of well-being; the terms have similar meanings, though euphoria may be considered more intense and excessive. Patients may laugh or tell jokes excessively or inappropriately, and they may be overly familiar with others. A related and more general concept is that of *disinhibition*, wherein patients may act impulsively, share too much personal information with others, or otherwise behave in ways that are socially inappropriate. Many of the behaviors I have already described, such as inappropriate sexual comments and behaviors, can represent disinhibition. Elation, euphoria, and disinhibition are hallmarks of the behavioral variant of FTD; these symptoms should also raise the possibility of traumatic brain injury (including subdural hematoma affecting the frontal lobes), stroke or tumor in the frontal lobes, and bipolar disorder.

A related construct is *pathological laughing and crying*, also known as pseudobulbar palsy, pseudobulbar affect, emotional incontinence, or involuntary emotional expression disorder. PLC has been described in patients with stroke, FTD, head injury, multiple sclerosis, and amyotrophic lateral sclerosis. Patients spontaneously cry (or, less commonly, laugh) without apparent precipitant and may be inconsolable. Pathological crying may differ from crying associated with depression in that patients with the former do not necessarily endorse feeling sad while they are crying—but the crying can be quite troubling to those around them. Pathological laughing may be puzzling and even offensive to others.

Alterations in Appetite and Eating

Patients with dementia can display a wide range of changes in appetite and eating, leading to a number of complications. Olfactory dysfunction is very common in AD and in LBD; this and an associated change in sense of taste can lead to decreased appetite and weight loss. As memory loss and executive dysfunction progress, patients with dementia may have more difficulty preparing meals and may resort to bland and repetitive diets. Concerns about the ability to cook safely may also arise. Patients may forget that they have eaten or drunk and demand to eat or drink again. Patients with FTD and other disorders affecting the frontal lobes may eat excessively, crave sweets or carbohydrates, or try to eat things that are not food. Some patients with FTD may express rigid preferences for specific foods. (Those caring for patients with FTD may describe such behaviors as obsessions or compulsions.) As dementia progresses, patients may develop dysphagia, leading to choking and aspiration; they may need prompting to chew and swallow food or they may try to put too much food in their mouth.

Acetylcholinesterase inhibitors (and many other classes of medications) can decrease appetite and result in weight loss. Weight loss is especially worrisome in older adults because they may lose much-needed muscle mass, which in turn can result in frailty and debilitation.

SUMMARY: IDENTIFYING BPSD AND THEIR SIGNIFICANCE

BPSD are common and potentially devastating to patients, their family members, and other caregivers. It is important for clinicians to have an understanding of how BPSD arise (see Figures 3–2 through 3–5) and their specific manifestations (see Table 3–2). Case Example 3–1 illustrates many of the points covered in this chapter.

Case Example 3–1: "He's Saying the Same Thing Over and Over Again—Please Give Him a Medication."

Mr. Wang is a 79-year-old man who was diagnosed with AD 5 years ago and who moved into an assisted living facility recently following the death of his wife. He has no relatives in the area and is estranged from his children. The staff members caring for Mr. Wang at this facility, which opened just 3 months ago and describes itself as a memory care unit, contact the primary care provider to ask for a medication to stop him from "saying the same thing over and over again." They seem well intentioned but also somewhat perplexed (and annoyed) by his behavior. They note that he uses the call button much more frequently than other residents, who tend to rest quietly in their rooms most of the time. Mr. Wang frequently calls out for his wife, even after they explain that she has died; sometimes they fib and say that she has stepped out for a few minutes and will return soon, but this does not seem to help. Mr. Wang asks for help toileting, even minutes after having used the restroom. Exasperated, one of the nurses says, "He won't be able to stay here if he keeps misbehaving like this."

A social worker at the primary care provider's office calls the staff of the assisted living facility to learn more. She validates their concern about the frequency of his behavior and also asks them to identify antecedents to the behavior as well as consequences. His repetitive statements seem to come most frequently around 5 P.M., when he also starts to become more forgetful and confused. The staff notes that he spends much of the morning in his room alone and is calm during those times. After lunch, he starts pacing around the hallways, asking to talk to staff and asking questions of other residents. The behavior is most incessant right before dinner time. The staff members patiently try to answer his questions, but doing so seems to lead to even more questions. At dinner, he calms down and seems to enjoy talking with the other residents at his table.

The social worker explains that, as predicted by the progressively lowered stress threshold model, Mr. Wang has less tolerance for stress in the evening. She suggests that a nap after lunch may help rejuvenate him and increase his stress threshold. The social worker also wonders what unmet need his behavior of repetitive statements may indicate. After exploring this topic together, the staff of the assisted living facility postulate that Mr. Wang is lonely—missing his deceased wife and his estranged children—and that his repetitive statements are an attempt to engage others and reduce his loneliness. The staff develops a plan to engage him more in social activities over the course of the day. They assign him the role of "door greeter," whereby (under supervision by staff) he can say hello to visitors as they enter the facility. Mr. Wang's repetitive statements subsequently decreased markedly.

KEY POINTS

- Approximately 90% of patients with AD experience clinically significant BPSD.

- Most of what is known about BPSD has been learned from studying patients with AD, but symptom similarities can be reasonably extrapolated to other causes of dementia.

- Depression is the most common of the BPSD in MCI and in mild dementia; delusions are the most common symptoms in moderate dementia; apathy and agitation are the most common symptoms in severe dementia.

- BPSD are distressing to both patients and caregivers and can lead to more frequent hospitalizations, earlier nursing home placement, increased mortality, abuse and neglect, caregiver depression and anxiety, and increased economic costs.

- Although there is no unified model of how BPSD arise, various approaches have been instructive, including 1) viewing BPSD as behaviors with antecedents and consequences; 2) recognizing that persons with dementia have progressively lower thresholds for stress, which leads to an increased risk of dysfunctional behaviors; 3) viewing BPSD as expressions of unmet needs of persons with dementia; 4) appreciating the interplay of medical factors, medication effects, psychological factors, and social factors in the emergence of BPSD; and 5) recognizing abnormalities in the functional networks involved in emotion regulation, and executive function.

- There are many different specific behavioral and psychological symptoms, each with its own implications:

  - Depression in dementia resembles major depressive episode, as described in DSM-5 (American Psychiatric Association 2013) but with more prominent irritability and social withdrawal. Anxiety is also quite common.

- Apathy differs from depression in that the former does not include psychological symptoms such as guilt, hopelessness, and worthlessness. Rather, lack of motivation is the core feature.
- Patients with dementia may make repetitive statements, scream, or say things that are sarcastic, derogatory, insulting, insensitive, or sexually inappropriate.
- Of great concern is physical aggression, which can be dangerous to patients and those around them. Wandering may also pose a significant threat to safety.
- Disturbances of the sleep-wake cycle are common, especially in AD and LBD. These problems include fragmented sleep-wake schedules, day-night reversal, sundowning, and REM sleep behavior disorder. Sleep disturbance among patients can take quite a toll on caregivers.
- Visual hallucinations and delusions are the hallmarks of LBD but can be present in any cause of dementia and can be quite distressing to patients and their caregivers.
- Disinhibition, elation, euphoria, and PLC arise most commonly in patients with disorders affecting the frontal lobes (specifically, FTD) but also in patients with stroke, traumatic brain injury, and other neurological conditions.
- Patients with dementia can experience a wide range of problems related to eating, including loss of the senses of taste and smell, loss of appetite, changes in dietary preferences, decreased ability to prepare meals (and do so safely), problems with chewing, dysphagia, choking, and aspiration.

RESOURCES FOR PATIENTS, FAMILIES, AND CAREGIVERS

Alzheimer's Association: Alzheimer's Disease Pocketcard. Free app for health-care provider that includes a wide range of educational material that can be shared with patients and family members. Available at the AppStore and Google play.

Alzheimer's Association: Stages and Behaviors. Chicago, IL, Alzheimer's Association, 2018. Available at: https://alz.org/help-support/caregiving/stages-behaviors. This web page provides an overview of BPSD and describes specific BPSD, including aggression and anger, anxiety and agitation, depression, hallucinations, repetition, sleep issues and sundowning, suspicions and delusions, and wandering.

Mace N, Rabins P: The 36-Hour Day: A Family Guide to Caring for People Who Have Alzheimer Disease, Related Dementias, and Memory Loss, 6th Edition. Baltimore, MD, Johns Hopkins University Press, 2017. This book, also listed as a resource in Chapter 2, provides comprehensive information for family members and other caregivers regarding BPSD and how to address them.

REFERENCES

Alexopoulos GS, Abrams RC, Young RC, Shamoian CA: Cornell Scale for Depression in Dementia. Biol Psychiatry 23(3):271–284, 1988 3337862

American Psychiatric Association: Diagnostic and Statistical Manual of Mental Disorders, 5th Edition. Arlington, VA, American Psychiatric Association, 2013

Bang J, Spina S, Miller BL: Frontotemporal dementia. Lancet 386(10004):1672–1682, 2015 26595641

Borsje P, Wetzels RB, Lucassen PL, et al: The course of neuropsychiatric symptoms in community-dwelling patients with dementia: a systematic review. Int Psychogeriatr 27(3):385–405, 2015 25403309

Boublay N, Schott AM, Krolak-Salmon P: Neuroimaging correlates of neuropsychiatric symptoms in Alzheimer's disease: a review of 20 years of research. Eur J Neurol 23(10):1500–1509, 2016 27435186

Casanova MF, Starkstein SE, Jellinger KA: Clinicopathological correlates of behavioral and psychological symptoms of dementia. Acta Neuropathol 122(2):117–135, 2011 21455688

Cheng S-T: Dementia caregiver burden: a research update and critical analysis. Curr Psychiatry Rep 19(9):64, 2017 28795386

Cummings J, Mintzer J, Brodaty H, et al: Agitation in cognitive disorders: International Psychogeriatric Association provisional consensus clinical and research definition. Int Psychogeriatr 27(1):7–17, 2015 25311499

Howell T: The Wisconsin Star Method: understanding and addressing complexity in geriatrics, in Geriatrics Models of Care: Bringing "Best Practice" to an Aging America, edited by Malone ML, Capezuti E, Palmer RM. New York, Springer International, 2015, pp 87–94

Jeste DV, Finkel SI: Psychosis of Alzheimer's disease and related dementias. Diagnostic criteria for a distinct syndrome. Am J Geriatr Psychiatry 8(1):29–34, 2000 10648292

Kales HC, Gitlin LN, Lyketsos CG: Management of neuropsychiatric symptoms of dementia in clinical settings: recommendations from a multidisciplinary expert panel. J Am Geriatr Soc 62(4):762–769, 2014 24635665

Kaufer DI, Cummings JL, Ketchel P, et al: Validation of the NPI-Q, a brief clinical form of the Neuropsychiatric Inventory. J Neuropsychiatry Clin Neurosci 12(2):233–239, 2000 11001602

Kovach CR, Noonan PE, Schlidt AM, et al: A model of consequences of need-driven, dementia-compromised behavior. J Nurs Scholarsh 37(2):134–140, discussion 140, 2005 15960057

McKeith IG, Boeve BF, Dickson DW, et al: Diagnosis and management of dementia with Lewy bodies: Fourth consensus report of the DLB Consortium. Neurology 89(1):88–100, 2017 28592453

McKhann G, Drachman D, Folstein M, et al: Clinical diagnosis of Alzheimer's disease: report of the NINCDS-ADRDA Work Group under the auspices of Department of Health and Human Services Task Force on Alzheimer's Disease. Neurology 34(7):939–944, 1984 6610841

Okura T, Plassman BL, Steffens DC, et al: Prevalence of neuropsychiatric symptoms and their association with functional limitations in older adults in the United States: the aging, demographics, and memory study. J Am Geriatr Soc 58(2):330–337, 2010 20374406

Olin JT, Schneider LS, Katz IR, et al: Provisional diagnostic criteria for depression of Alzheimer disease. Am J Geriatr Psychiatry 10(2):125–128, 2002 11925273

Osborne H, Simpson J, Stokes G: The relationship between pre-morbid personality and challenging behaviour in people with dementia: a systematic review. Aging Ment Health 14(5):503–515, 2010 20480417

Panza F, Frisardi V, Seripa D, et al: Apolipoprotein E genotypes and neuropsychiatric symptoms and syndromes in late-onset Alzheimer's disease. Ageing Res Rev 11(1):87–103, 2012 21763789

Polenick CA, Struble LM, Stanislawski B, et al: "The filter is kind of broken": family caregivers' attributions about behavioral and psychological symptoms of dementia. Am J Geriatr Psychiatry 26(5):548–556, 2018 29373300

Rosenberg PB, Nowrangi MA, Lyketsos CG: Neuropsychiatric symptoms in Alzheimer's disease: what might be associated brain circuits? Mol Aspects Med 43–44:25–37, 2015 26049034

Sallim AB, Sayampanathan AA, Cuttilan A, et al: Prevalence of mental health disorders among caregivers of patients with Alzheimer disease. J Am Med Dir Assoc 16(12):1034–1041, 2015 26593303

Seyfried LS, Kales HC, Ignacio RV, et al: Predictors of suicide in patients with dementia. Alzheimers Dement 7(6):567–573, 2011 22055973

Sheikh JI, Yesavage JA: Geriatric Depression Scale (GDS): Recent evidence and development of a shorter version. Clin Gerontol 5:165–173, 1986

Smith M, Gerdner LA, Hall GR, et al: History, development, and future of the progressively lowered stress threshold: a conceptual model for dementia care. J Am Geriatr Soc 52(10):1755–1760, 2004 15450057

Spitzer RL, Kroenke K, William JR: Validation and utility of a self-report version of PRIME-MD: the PHQ primary care study: primary care evaluation of mental disorders: Patient Health Questionnaire. JAMA 282(18):1737–1744, 1999 10568646

Suzuki R, Goebert D, Ahmed I, Lu B: Folk and biological perceptions of dementia among Asian ethnic minorities in Hawaii. Am J Geriatr Psychiatry 23(6):589–595, 2015 24801608

Teri L, Logsdon RG, Weiner MF, et al: Treatment for agitation in dementia patients: a behavior management approach. Psychotherapy 35:436–443, 1998

Tiel C, Sudo FK, Alves GS, et al: Neuropsychiatric symptoms in vascular cognitive impairment: a systematic review. Dement Neuropsychol 9(3):230–236, 2015 29213966

Zhao Q-F, Tan L, Wang H-F, et al: The prevalence of neuropsychiatric symptoms in Alzheimer's disease: systematic review and meta-analysis. J Affect Disord 190:264–271, 2016 26540080

CHAPTER 4

ASSESSMENT OF BEHAVIORAL AND PSYCHOLOGICAL SYMPTOMS OF DEMENTIA

Prior to developing a plan to help a patient with behavioral and psychological symptoms of dementia (BPSD), one should identify the underlying cause of dementia because this may influence both the understanding and the treatment of BPSD. Next, a careful exploration of the BPSD should be undertaken, characterizing each symptom, its frequency, and its intensity. The clinician should examine antecedents and consequences of the behaviors because these may provoke or reinforce symptoms. The next step is identifying medical and environmental causes that may be contributing. Various frameworks are available for structuring this process, such as the Targeted Interdisciplinary Model for Evaluation and Treatment of Neuropsychiatric Symptoms (TIME; Lichtwarck et al. 2017) and "describe, investigate, create, evaluate" (DICE; Kales et al. 2014). When the safety of patients and those around them is a concern, the process of assessment may need to be accelerated or abbreviated—but still needs to take place.

DIAGNOSIS OF UNDERLYING DEMENTIA

As discussed extensively in Chapter 1, an important step in understanding and addressing BPSD is determining the etiology of dementia. In the midst of a crisis precipitated by BPSD, this may not be immediately feasible, but eventually the correct diagnosis should be established. In some instances, it may not even be clear that a patient has dementia until BPSD have emerged—thus necessitating a diagnostic evaluation of dementia during or after the assessment of BPSD. See Tables 1–1 and 1–2 in Chapter 1 for an overview of the causes of dementia (major neurocognitive disorder) and for the components of assessing dementia, respectively.

Briefly, the most salient causes of dementia to consider in the context of assessing BPSD are Lewy body disease (LBD) and frontotemporal dementia (FTD). LBD, which includes both Parkinson disease dementia (initially a motor disorder, followed by cognitive and psychiatric impairment) and dementia with Lewy bodies (primarily a neurocognitive disorder, with associated psychiatric and motor involvement), can include prominent psychiatric symptoms, including vivid visual hallucinations, delusions, anxiety, and sleep disturbance due to rapid eye movement (REM) sleep behavior disorder; furthermore, patients with LBD are exquisitely sensitive to the extrapyramidal side effects of antipsychotic medications. The core features of the behavioral variant of FTD include verbal aggression, physical aggression, disinhibition, apathy, and disturbances in appetite and eating. FTD typically afflicts younger patients (ages 45–64 years). The new onset of behavioral and cognitive impairment in a patient in this age group should trigger a search for FTD.

The most common cause of dementia is Alzheimer's disease (AD), which manifests as a slowly progressive loss of memory and other cognitive domains, with concomitant loss in functioning. Most patients with AD will experience BPSD at some point over the course of their illness, and most literature about BPSD comes from studies of patients with AD.

Depending on the location of cerebrovascular lesions, patients with vascular dementia may manifest various BPSD, including apathy, depression, and hallucinations. Mixed dementias (AD plus LBD, or AD plus vascular dementia) are also common, and patients present with a blend of symptoms of each type of dementia.

Delirium may complicate dementia and may manifest as the acute onset of BPSD. I discuss conducting an evaluation of delirium in the section "Biological Factors" later in this chapter. Although I have been referring to BPSD in the context of dementia (major neurocognitive disorder), it is important to recognize that patients with mild neurocognitive disorder (defined as cognitive impairment without significant functional impairment), also known as mild cognitive impairment (MCI), also commonly experience BPSD, especially symptoms of depression and anxiety.

SPECIFYING AND CHARACTERIZING BPSD

Typically, a clinical encounter related to BPSD begins with a patient, family member, or other caregiver reporting a symptom of concern. To appropriately address BPSD, it is essential that the clinician first obtain a detailed understanding of the presentation. This requires both fully exploring the symptom of concern and, because BPSD often co-occur, screening for other symptoms. If there is an imminent risk of harm to the patient or to those around the patient, a detailed analysis may need to be delayed until safety can be assured.

For each symptom of concern (e.g., wandering, verbal aggression), the clinician should elicit a detailed description of the behavior—specifically the timing, severity, antecedents, consequences, and history—as detailed in Table 4–1.

When working with the staff of a facility, a form similar to the one in Figure 4–1 could be helpful for structuring this process. Alternatively, the clinician could ask a facility to track specific symptoms, including their frequency and severity, or could ask to review documentation if the facility already has it. The staff of a facility or family members may refer to *sundowning* (or "sundowners")—that is, worsening of symptoms during the late afternoon or evening; though this is useful information about the timing of symptoms, it is still important to get more specific information about the nature of the symptoms.

When multiple symptoms are present, it may not be possible to address all of them at or around the same time. Therefore, I would recommend asking the patient or caregiver to rank-order the symptoms, with the idea that more consequential or potentially dangerous symptoms should be addressed first. For example, wandering (which could be dangerous, for instance, if a patient wanders out of the house in inclement weather) would take priority over verbal repetitions (which may be annoying but not dangerous).

When there is one particularly distressing or dangerous symptom present, patients and their caregivers may not notice or report all of the BPSD that are present. Another symptom may in fact help explain the symptom of concern. For example, a caregiver reports that a nursing home resident becomes physically aggressive at dinner; upon further exploration, it turns out that the patient has developed paranoid ideation about one of the other residents who shares the same dinner table. Table 4–2 presents a recommended approach to screening for all BPSD.

Collecting comprehensive and consistent information about the behaviors of a patient with dementia can be a challenge. Caregivers may have difficulty recalling details, especially if they are depressed, anxious, sleep deprived, or experiencing caregiver burnout. In an institutional setting, many caregivers are usually involved, and each one may witness some or none of the concerning symptoms. Problems with communication may

TABLE 4–1. Characterizing a behavioral or psychological symptom of dementia

Characteristic	Questions to ask
Timing	How often does the symptom occur? When the symptom arises, how long does it last? How long has this symptom been present (i.e., when was the onset of the symptom)?
Severity	Is this behavior imminently dangerous to the patient or to others (family members, other caregivers, other residents of the patient's facility)? If not imminently dangerous, could it escalate and become imminently dangerous? Does the behavior pose other risks (e.g., are caregivers refusing to come into the home, is the patient at risk of losing housing)? Is the behavior contributing to burnout on the part of caregivers? Is the behavior interfering with appropriate care of the patient? Is the behavior preventing the patient from participating in activities? Is the behavior causing the patient distress?
Antecedents	Do there appear to be any precipitants to the behavior? If so, does the behavior occur *only* when a precipitant occurs, or can it occur at other times? Does the behavior *always* follow the precipitant? Does the behavior occur at a particular time of day (e.g., late afternoon or early evening, as seen in sundowning)? Does the behavior occur only with a particular caregiver? Was there any apparent trigger or change prior to the onset of the behavior? Is there any other apparent pattern to the behavior?
Consequences	How do family members and other caregivers respond to the symptom? What impact does the response in turn have on the patient? Is it possible that through their responses, caregivers are either unwittingly reinforcing or exacerbating the behavior? Conversely, have caregivers found a response that has been effective at reducing the frequency, duration, or severity of the behavior?
History	Is this a new behavior? If the behavior is not new, is it different in severity or quality from prior instances of the behavior?

cause each party to have incomplete information; other barriers can include turnover of staff and deficiencies in the training of staff. Given their cognitive impairments and psychiatric symptoms (e.g., delusions), patients themselves may have very different perspectives on the reported symptoms. All of

---

**CONCERN ABOUT THE BEHAVIOR
OF A RESIDENT WITH DEMENTIA**

Please use this form to report your concern about the behavior of one of your residents who is also our patient.
If the resident or others are in imminent danger, call 911.

Resident's name: _____   DOB: ___ / ___ / _____

Name of person
completing this form: _____   Phone: _____   Fax: _____

BEHAVIORS
List the specific behaviors you
are concerned about: _____

How long has this been going on? ___ days / weeks / months   How frequent is it? _____

Does anything seem to make the behaviors
better or worse, including time of day?   _____

What interventions have been tried,
including PRN medications?   _____

What has been the effect of these interventions? _____

MEDICAL ISSUES
List any medication changes in the last month
(new, discontinued, increased, decreased):   _____

List any new medical symptoms (for example,
cough, falls, pain, frequent urination):   _____

List any recent lab tests (for example, urinalysis):
including dates and results: _____

COORDINATION OF CARE
Does the patient have an activated Health Care Power of Attorney or guardian? __ yes __ no

     If "yes," have you discussed your concerns with her/him?   __ yes __ no

                                                        → If "no," please do so now

Have you contacted any other physicians about this behavior?   __ yes __ no

     If "yes," list who, when, and the response: _____

FIGURE 4–1.   Form for reporting behavioral and psychological symptoms of dementia.

I use this form to aid in the collection of information from caregiving staff at assisted living facilities and long-term care facilities. The form helps staff specify the behavioral and psychological symptoms of concern, antecedents to the behavior, and consequences of the behavior, including how staff responded and the outcome of this response.

DOB = date of birth; PRN = as needed.

TABLE 4–2. Screening for specific behavioral and psychological symptoms of dementia

Symptom	What to ask patients	What to ask caregivers
Depression	Have you been feeling sad or down recently? Have you given up activities or hobbies you used to enjoy? Do you feel hopeless, guilty, or worthless? Do you feel like it would be better to be dead than alive? Have you developed any plans to harm yourself or end your life?	Has he or she been more withdrawn or less active recently? Has he or she appeared down or tearful? Has he or she talked about wanting to die or to hurt himself or herself?
Apathy	Are you less interested in activities or hobbies than you used to be? What do you make of others' concerns about you?	Does he or she seem to be less concerned about his or her situation or about others or about news or events? Is he or she less affectionate? Is he or she less likely to start or participate in conversations? Do you find yourself frustrated by his or her being less concerned?
Verbal aggression and other vocalizations	Are you in pain? Are you worried that something bad is going to happen to you?	Does he or she say anything out of character, offensive, or inappropriate? Does he or she ask the same question or say the same thing over and over again? Does he or she yell or scream?
Physical aggression, agitation, and other aberrant motor behaviors	I have heard that you sometimes [name behavior]—can you say why?	Is he or she pushing, grabbing, scratching, hitting, kicking, or biting others? Is he or she hitting or throwing objects? Is he or she interfering with the care of others? Do you feel unsafe?

TABLE 4–2. Screening for specific behavioral and psychological symptoms of dementia *(continued)*

Symptom	What to ask patients	What to ask caregivers
Refusing medications or assistance with activities of daily living	I have heard that you sometimes do not take all your medications (or do not want help when others offer it)—can you say why?	Are there pills left in pill box at the end of the week? Does he or she spit out or appear to cheek pills? Does he or she get upset when help is offered or refuse help?
Wandering	Why are you leaving the house? Is something scaring you at home? Are you looking for someone?	Does he or she attempt to leave the house/facility? Does he or she say why?
Disturbances of sleep-wake cycle	Do you have any trouble falling asleep? Do you have any trouble staying asleep? Do you wake up too early or too late? Do you nap during the daytime?	What time does he or she go to bed? Does he or she have trouble falling asleep? Is he or she restless or up at night? If so, what does he or she do (yell, kick, wander)? Does he or she snore loudly or appear to stop breathing? Do behaviors get worse in the late afternoon or evening? How are you sleeping?
Anxiety and irritability	Are you worried that something bad is going to happen to you? Are you afraid of falling? Are you afraid to leave the house? Do you get upset easily?	Is he or she afraid to be left alone? Does he or she follow you around the house? Is he or she more irritable or easily upset?

TABLE 4–2. Screening for specific behavioral and psychological symptoms of dementia *(continued)*

Symptom	What to ask patients	What to ask caregivers
Delusions and hallucinations	Do you feel like someone is trying to hurt or kill you? Do you feel like someone is stealing from you? When you are by yourself, do you hear any voices talking to you or about you? Do you see any creatures or strangers in the house?	Does he or she accuse you of stealing from him or her, being unfaithful to him or her, or not being who you say you are? Does he or she talk about there being animals or people in the house who are not there? Does he or she seem to be listening to sounds that are not there?
Elation, euphoria, and disinhibition	Do you feel happier than usual? Do you do or say anything that you later regret?	Is he or she in a much better mood than usual? Is he or she telling too many jokes or jokes that are inappropriate?
Pathological laughing and crying	Do you ever find yourself crying even when you don't feel sad? Do you ever find yourself laughing even when you don't feel happy?	Does he or she start crying (or laughing) out of the blue without a clear cause?
Alterations in appetite and eating	Has your appetite changed? Have you lost or gained weight? Do your clothes fit any differently recently?	Is he or she eating less or eating more? Has he or she lost or gained weight? Is he or she eating anything unusual? Is he or she having trouble swallowing, choking, or coughing during meals?

this can lead to a Rashomon effect, thereby requiring the clinician to piece together a coherent narrative from conflicting information. Asking the primary caregiver (or, in an institutional setting, the staff member most familiar with the patient) to complete a form like the one presented earlier in Figure 4–1 can help address some of these concerns. To get more granular data—namely, the presence of specific behaviors for each hour of the day over the course of a week—the clinician can ask a caregiver to complete the form in Figure 4–2; this form could also be used to track responses to interventions. Long-term care facilities may already have such forms in place, in which case the clinician could ask staff members to share a copy of their data. Over time, educating the patient and caregivers regarding the presentation of BPSD can eventually lead to more accurate and actionable information.

A structured model can be helpful both as an educational tool and a clinical tool. For example, the TIME tool has been found to reduce agitation in nursing home residents with dementia (Lichtwarck et al. 2018). The TIME approach includes three phases:

1. *Registration and assessment phase:* Clinician examines the patient, obtains previous medical records, collects background information, and registers BPSD in detailed 24-hour records.
2. *Guided reflection phase:* One or more case conferences are held to apply a "cognitive problem-solving method" to each BPSD, which includes assessed facts, interpretation, staff members' emotions/reactions, action to take, and evaluation.
3. *Action and evaluation phase:* Agreed-upon actions are implemented and evaluated.

An alternate approach has been labeled DICE (Kales et al. 2014), an acronym for the four major steps involved in addressing BPSD:

- *Describe* the problematic behavior.
- *Investigate* possible causes of the behavior.
- *Create* a treatment plan.
- *Evaluate* the outcome of this plan.

Of most relevance to the current discussion is the "describe" component of the model: the caregiver describes the context (who, what, when, and where) of the behavior, the social and physical environment, the patient perspective, and the degree of distress to the patient and caregiver. Both TIME and DICE are manualized interventions that can be used in training facility and social services staff. See the section "Etiological Models of BPSD" in Chapter 3 for a discussion of the Wisconsin Star Method as another structured approach.

The "American Psychiatric Association Practice Guideline on the Use of Antipsychotics to Treat Agitation or Psychosis in Patients With Dementia" (Reus et al. 2016) recommends the following:

LOG OF CONCERNING BEHAVIORS

Patient's name: _____   DOB: ___ /___ /_____

Reporter's name: _____   Phone: _____ Fax: _____

Here is a list of behaviors that could be a source of concern or danger:			Pick the most common or concerning behaviors, and assign each one a code:	
Sleep problem	Hallucinations	Euphoria	A =	D =
Agitation or aggression	Delusions or paranoia	Restlessness or wandering	B =	E =
Anxiety	Apathy or indifference	Irritability or lability		
Disinhibition	Depression		C =	F =

For each day and hour that there is a concerning behavior(s), write down the code(s), and describe what happened.

Date: __ / __

7a	8	9	10	11	12p	1	2	3	4	5	6	7	8	9	10	11	12a	1	2	3	4	5	6

Comments:

Date: __ / __

7a	8	9	10	11	12p	1	2	3	4	5	6	7	8	9	10	11	12a	1	2	3	4	5	6

Comments:

Date: __ / __

7a	8	9	10	11	12p	1	2	3	4	5	6	7	8	9	10	11	12a	1	2	3	4	5	6

Comments:

Date: __ / __

7a	8	9	10	11	12p	1	2	3	4	5	6	7	8	9	10	11	12a	1	2	3	4	5	6

Comments:

Date: __ / __

7a	8	9	10	11	12p	1	2	3	4	5	6	7	8	9	10	11	12a	1	2	3	4	5	6

Comments:

Date: __ / __

7a	8	9	10	11	12p	1	2	3	4	5	6	7	8	9	10	11	12a	1	2	3	4	5	6

Comments:

Date: __ / __ (month / date)

7a	8	9	10	11	12p	1	2	3	4	5	6	7	8	9	10	11	12a	1	2	3	4	5	6

Comments:

FIGURE 4–2. Form for logging behavioral and psychological symptoms of dementia over time.

This form could be used by the staff of a facility or, with some explanation, a family member caring for a person with dementia.

DOB = date of birth.

Source. Adapted from Lichtwarck et al. 2017.

- Assessing the type, frequency, severity, pattern, and timing of symptoms
- Assessing patients with dementia "for pain and other potentially modifiable contributors to symptoms as well as for factors, such as the subtype of dementia, that may influence choices of treatment" (p. 544)
- Assessing patients using quantitative measures—that is, rating scales

Rating scales have been used primarily in research to determine the frequency and severity of BPSD and to measure the effect of interventions on BPSD. Often, predetermined cutoffs are established as criteria for inclusion or exclusion in intervention trials; this leads to the often-seen experience that interventions work better in research trials in which only significantly severe behavior is addressed and patients improve significantly but continue to have mild severity and less frequent BPSD. In many clinical practices that attempt to use the same intervention (pharmacological or nonpharmacological) for much milder and infrequent behaviors, the intervention may not seem to work because BPSD interventions seldom completely eliminate the symptom.

In a clinical setting, rating scales may also be of value but can be cumbersome to administer. The most widely used rating scales to assess the full range of BPSD are the Neuropsychiatric Inventory (NPI) and its clinical variant, the NPI–Questionnaire (NPI-Q; Kaufer et al. 2000). The NPI-Q covers 12 domains of BPSD, starting with a screening question (e.g., for delusions, "Does the patient have false beliefs, such as thinking that others are stealing from him/her or planning to harm him/her in some way?"); if the screen is positive, the informant is then asked to rate the severity (mild, moderate, severe) of the symptom and the distress that the informant experiences as a result of the symptom (not distressing at all, minimal, mild, moderate, severe, extreme or very severe). In the NPI–Nursing Home Version (NPI-NH), the screening question for each of the 12 BPSD domains is followed by several "subquestions" to further characterize the symptoms, a frequency rating (rarely, sometimes, often, very often), a severity rating (mild, moderate, severe), and a rating of "occupational disruptiveness" ("How much does this behavior upset you and/or create more work for you?") (Wood et al. 2000). Alternatives to the NPI and its variants include the Cohen-Mansfield Agitation Inventory (Cohen-Mansfield 1986) and the Behavioral Pathology in Alzheimer's Disease (BEHAVE-AD) rating scale (Reisberg et al. 1987).

Rating scales are commonly used to screen for and assess depression in older adults. Unfortunately, the Patient Health Questionnaire–9 (PHQ-9) and the Geriatric Depression Scale (GDS) are not reliable for assessing patients who have significant cognitive impairment. An empirically validated alternative for older adults with cognitive impairment is the Cornell Scale for Depression in Dementia (CSDD), which takes about 30 minutes to administer and involves a clinician interviewing the patient and a caregiver (Alexopoulos et al. 1988). The CSDD is available online and may be used with permission from the author.

The Rating Anxiety in Dementia (RAID) involves a clinician interviewing both the patient and a caregiver to assess the presence and severity (absent, mild or intermittent, moderate, severe) of 18 symptoms of anxiety in four categories: worry, apprehension and vigilance, motor tension, and autonomic hyperactivity (Shankar et al. 1999). Phobias and panic attacks are also assessed but are not tallied in the total score.

BIOLOGICAL FACTORS

I discuss neurobiological correlates of BPSD in Chapter 3 (see the section "Etiological Models of BPSD"), but these do not necessarily inform the diagnostic evaluation. A number of physiological conditions should be considered, screened for, and ruled out when determining what might have caused or what might otherwise be contributing to BPSD. Broadly, these include metabolic disturbances, infectious diseases, and central nervous system insults, which are detailed in Table 4–3 along with recommended evaluations. Other conditions such as constipation, urinary retention, dehydration, malnutrition, vision loss, hearing loss, and pain may also cause or contribute to BPSD. (See the section "Identifying and Addressing Pain" in Chapter 2 for a detailed discussion of the assessment of pain in patients with dementia.) Clinicians should maintain a high index of suspicion for sleep disorders such as obstructive sleep apnea, restless legs syndrome, and REM sleep behavior disorder.

Any number of infections that would not necessarily cause neuropsychiatric symptoms in younger adults and healthy older adults may manifest as BPSD in patients with dementia. For example, mental status changes are the presenting symptom in approximately half of long-term care residents hospitalized for pneumonia (Jump et al. 2018). The site of infection may be difficult to discern. For example, I have seen a case of an older patient with a dental abscess manifesting as subacute delirium; an astute primary care provider thought to examine the patient's oral cavity. Note that leukocytosis may not occur in older adults with infection, so a normal white blood cell count does not rule out infection.

There is some controversy about whether or not a urinary tract infection (UTI) alone can precipitate delirium or BPSD. Long-standing teaching

TABLE 4–3. Medical causes of behavioral and psychological symptoms of dementia (BPSD) (and delirium) and recommended evaluations

Category	Medical condition	Comments and suggested evaluation
Metabolic disturbances	Hyponatremia or hypernatremia, hypocalcemia or hypercalcemia, hypomagnesemia or hypermagnesemia	Medications (diuretics, antidepressants), dehydration, and alcohol use may cause electrolyte disturbances. *Check serum electrolytes in all patients with new or altered BPSD.*
	Hypoglycemia or hyperglycemia	Maintain high index of suspicion in patients with diabetes mellitus, especially if treated with insulin. *Check serum glucose or finger-stick glucose in all patients with new or altered BPSD.*
	Acute kidney injury	Dehydration and chronic kidney disease place patients at risk of acute kidney injury. *Check BUN and creatinine in all patients with new or altered BPSD. Creatinine may not be accurate in older adults, so glomerular filtration rate should be calculated.*
	Hypoxia, hypercarbia	Maintain high index of suspicion in patients with COPD. *Check pulse oximetry if hypoxia is suspected. In rare cases, arterial blood gases may be necessary to rule out hypercarbia.*
	Hepatic encephalopathy	Maintain high index of suspicion in patients with hepatic disease or on medications that can cause liver damage (valproate, duloxetine). *Check bilirubin, transaminases, and perhaps ammonia if patient has history of hepatic disease.*

TABLE 4–3. Medical causes of behavioral and psychological symptoms of dementia (BPSD) (and delirium) and recommended evaluations *(continued)*

Category	Medical condition	Comments and suggested evaluation
Metabolic disturbances *(continued)*	Thiamine deficiency (Wernicke's encephalopathy)	Patients with history of severe alcohol use are at risk of thiamine deficiency. Other vitamin deficiencies (e.g., B_{12}) are unlikely to manifest as new BPSD. *Check thiamine level, if condition is suspected.*
	Hypothyroidism or hyperthyroidism	Unless severe, these are unlikely to manifest as new BPSD, except depression. However, ruling out thyroid dysfunction is a standard of evaluating dementia. *If not done in the last year, check thyroid-stimulating hormone.*
Infectious diseases	Urinary tract infection	See text for discussion. *Check urinalysis with microscopy in all patients with new or altered BPSD; if evidence of infection, check urine culture. Do not treat empirically with antibiotics.*
	Meningitis or encephalitis	Patients will typically be very ill (fever, obtundation, other systemic signs), but this is unlikely to be a cause of BPSD. *If condition is suspected, then hospitalization and appropriate evaluation are indicated.*
	Other infections	See text for discussion. *Evaluation depends on suspected site of infection (e.g., chest X-ray for suspected pneumonia). Checking a CBC is reasonable, but older adults with infection may not have leukocytosis.*

TABLE 4–3. Medical causes of behavioral and psychological symptoms of dementia (BPSD) (and delirium) and recommended evaluations *(continued)*

Category	Medical condition	Comments and suggested evaluation
Central nervous system insults	Cerebrovascular accident, ischemic or hemorrhagic stroke	Sudden onset or change in cognition or BPSD may be due to stroke. Hemorrhagic stroke should be detectable by CT; ischemic stroke may require MRI. *Order head CT or brain MRI, if condition is suspected.*
	Subdural hematoma	Patients with dementia are at risk of falling and head injury, which may occur without being witnessed. *Order head CT if condition is suspected.*
	Epileptic seizure or postictal state	This should be suspected if brief periods of confusion, garbled speech, or unusual behavior without clear precipitant is described. *Order neurological consultation and consider EEG, if condition is suspected.*
	Traumatic brain injury	*No specific testing is indicated—diagnosis will depend on history and caregiver report.*
Other	Constipation, urinary retention, dehydration, malnutrition	*Except perhaps for BUN and creatinine, no specific testing is indicated—diagnosis will depend on history and caregiver report.*
	Vision loss, hearing loss	Both are very common in older adults. Eyeglasses and hearing aids are easily lost. *Diagnosis will depend on history and caregiver report.*

TABLE 4–3.   Medical causes of behavioral and psychological
symptoms of dementia (BPSD) (and delirium) and
recommended evaluations *(continued)*

Category	Medical condition	Comments and suggested evaluation
Other *(continued)*	Pain	This is very common; patients may not be able to report pain, which may manifest as BPSD instead. See section "Identifying and Addressing Pain" in Chapter 2 for further discussion. *Specifically assess for pain; consider the use of rating scale, such as PAINAD.*
	OSA, RLS, RBD	OSA may contribute to depression and apathy. RLS and RBD may contribute to agitated behavior at night. RBD is prevalent in patients with Lewy body disease. *RLS and RBD are clinical diagnoses; order polysomnography to diagnose OSA.*

Note.   BUN=blood urea nitrogen; CBC=complete blood count; COPD=chronic obstructive pulmonary disease; CT=computed tomography; EEG=electroencephalogram; MRI=magnetic resonance imaging; OSA=obstructive sleep apnea; PAINAD=Pain Assessment in Advanced Dementia; RBD=rapid eye movement sleep behavior disorder; RLS=restless legs syndrome.

has held that this is possible and perhaps even common. However, some researchers have cast doubt on this purported relationship, arguing that many nursing home residents with indwelling catheters (and even some without catheters) will have chronic microbial colonization without active infection and that routine cultures then confuse this with symptomatic infection and lead to excessive, inappropriate antibiotic use (D'Agata et al. 2013). Therefore, most guidelines argue that a UTI should be considered only if there are also other signs or symptoms, such as recent onset of dysuria, urgency, frequency, or urethral purulence (van Buul et al. 2018). My recommendation would be to check a urinalysis as part of the delirium/BPSD evaluation; if the urinalysis suggests infection (pyuria, presence of leukocyte esterase), then urine should be submitted for culture to see if a pathogen that could be responsible for UTI (e.g., *Escherichia coli*) grows. An antibiotic should not be prescribed empirically; rather, one should wait for the result of the urine culture.

The acute onset of new BPSD should raise suspicion for delirium. Whereas dementia typically includes slow, steady decline in cognition, delirium manifests as the sudden onset (within hours to days) of mental status changes. Sometimes, what is described as sundowning may in fact represent the waxing and waning mental status of delirium. Delirium is often multifactorial, with contributors including medical conditions, medication and substance use or withdrawal, and environmental factors.

The relationship between dementia, delirium, and BPSD is complex (Höltta et al. 2011). Dementia is a risk factor for delirium; delirium in turn seems to exacerbate cognitive decline, as evidenced by patients with dementia who do not return to their cognitive baseline following an episode of delirium. The fluctuating cognition seen in dementia with Lewy bodies can appear quite similar to the acute onset of confusion seen in delirium. Patients with dementia take longer to recover from delirium than do patients without dementia; the former may have subtle signs of delirium even weeks after onset. Most patients with BPSD will not simultaneously be delirious, whereas most patients with delirium superimposed on dementia will also have some behavioral and/or psychological symptoms (Figure 4–3). A patient could have delirium without associated BPSD, as in the case of a patient who is lethargic or obtunded due to delirium, and therefore unable to manifest any behavioral disturbance or emotional symptoms.

A clinician can use the Confusion Assessment Method (CAM) to make the diagnosis of delirium (Figure 4–4). The positive predictive value (i.e., probability that the patient has delirium if the CAM is positive) is 91%–94%; the negative predictive value (i.e., the probability the patient does not have delirium if the CAM is negative) is 90%–100% (Inouye et al. 1990). Note that the *Diagnostic and Statistical Manual of Mental Disorders* has changed since the CAM was developed; for example, DSM-5 (American Psychiatric Association 2013) also requires "an additional disturbance in cognition (e.g., memory deficit, disorientation, language, visuospatial ability, or perception)" (p. 596). The impact of the subtle differences between the CAM and DSM-5 on the diagnosis of delirium is not clear. The workup of delirium is nearly identical to that of BPSD, as detailed in Table 4–2. The emphasis of treatment is on addressing the etiology of delirium (e.g., treating the infection causing the delirium).

Finally, there is the practical matter of how to conduct an appropriate diagnostic investigation in a patient who may not be able to cooperate with

Behavioral and Psychological Symptoms of Dementia

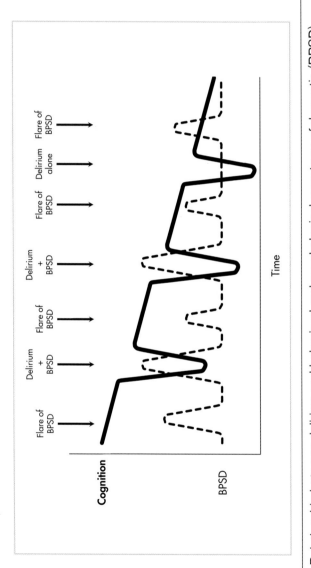

FIGURE 4-3. Relationship between delirium and behavioral and psychological symptoms of dementia (BPSD).

Cognition (*bold curve*) gradually declines over the course of dementia. Dementia is a risk factor for delirium. Delirium manifests as a sudden, sharp decrease in cognition, as illustrated by the three valleys in the cognition curve. Cognition tends not to return to baseline following an episode of delirium. BPSD (*dashed curve*) can occur independently of episodes of delirium or may be due to delirium. The sudden onset of new BPSD should raise concern for the possibility of delirium. Although delirium that is not complicated by BPSD occurs less commonly, it is possible (*third valley in the cognition curve*).

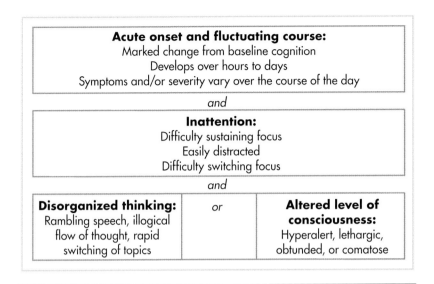

FIGURE 4–4. Confusion Assessment Method (CAM).

CAM is a screening test for delirium that incorporates the diagnostic criteria for delirium. If the patient has acute and fluctuating course *and* inattention *and* either disorganized thinking or altered level of consciousness, the CAM is positive, and there is a high likelihood the patient has delirium.

Source. Adapted from Inouye et al. 1990.

the recommended tests, including phlebotomy, urine collection, and (in some instances) neuroimaging. Attempting to collect blood from a patient who is physically aggressive may put both the patient and the medical staff in harm's way. The clinician may have to delay some or all of the evaluation and begin empirical treatment based on a preliminary understanding of the situation.

MEDICATIONS, ALCOHOL, AND OTHER SUBSTANCES

The onset of new BPSD or a marked change in preexisting BPSD should lead the clinician to scrutinize the patient's medication regimen, including over-the-counter (OTC) medications, dietary supplements, and complementary and alternative medicine interventions. The prevalence of use of OTC medications and supplements by older adults to relieve symptoms is quite high—in one sample, 89% and 26%, respectively (Arcury et al. 2012); in the same sample, 70% used vitamins, 60% used supplements, and 32%

used herbs to try to prevent illness (Arcury et al. 2015). Many medications and substances can contribute to BPSD (Table 4–4), and discontinuing offending agents should lead to improvement in BPSD.

For residents of long-term care facilities, a medication administration record should be available, listing both scheduled and as-needed medications, including the date, time, and reason for each as-needed use. It can be challenging for the clinician to obtain a comprehensive list of medications for patients living at home or residing in other settings where they take their own medications. It has been recommended that a caregiver bring in bottles of all medications (prescription, OTC, and supplements) for the clinician to review (Kales et al. 2014). The clinician should also consider drug-drug interactions; I would recommend entering all medications a patient is taking into a computerized application designed to identify such interactions. Using the Beers Criteria for Potentially Inappropriate Medication Use in Older Adults (commonly called the Beers list) may also be helpful (American Geriatrics Society 2019 Beers Criteria Update Expert Panel 2019). Clinicians should be especially alert to the addition of any new medications or changes of dosages or timing of current medications.

I review the deleterious effects of alcohol in patients with dementia in the section "Other Causes of Dementia" in Chapter 1. The rate of binge drinking in the United States skyrocketed from 2005/2006 to 2013/2014 to 22% for men and 9% for women age 50 years and older (Han and Moore 2018). Approximately 5% of older adults assessed in 2012–2013 in the United States had used cannabis in the past year, a relative increase of 58% from 2006–2007 (Han and Moore 2018). Although the effect of cannabis use on BPSD is unclear, a small trial of patients with AD found that the top five side effects of cannabis were anxiety, emotional lability, tiredness, somnolence, and euphoria (Ahmed et al. 2015). Concern has also arisen about cannabis use being associated with stroke and cognitive impairment (Han and Moore 2018). Cocaine may also cause stroke but is used rarely by older adults (0.4% of those age 50 years and older reported use in the past year). Finally, the opioid use epidemic has not spared older adults, with 1.4% of U.S. adults age 50 years and older using opioids nonmedically (Han and Moore 2018). In other words, clinicians should carefully assess patients with BPSD for use of alcohol and other substances.

PSYCHOLOGICAL FACTORS

Persons with dementia are psychological beings—with beliefs, values, insights, desires, hopes, urges, emotions, and a need for meaning and pur-

TABLE 4–4. Medications and other substances that can cause behavioral and psychological symptoms of dementia (BPSD)

Medications or substance	Comments and recommendations
Alcohol	At-risk alcohol use is fairly common among older adults. Either alcohol use or withdrawal could manifest as BPSD. Patients may drink more alcohol than reported. *Assess all patients with BPSD for alcohol use.*
Anticholinergic medications	Many categories of medications have anticholinergic properties, including medications for urinary incontinence, over-the-counter antihistamines for insomnia and allergic rhinitis, tricyclic antidepressants, and paroxetine. Anticholinergic side effects include sedation, confusion, hallucinations, falls, constipation, and urinary retention.
Antidepressants	Antidepressants (especially SSRIs and SNRIs) can cause hyponatremia, which in turn may cause BPSD. Antidepressants may paradoxically worsen depression or anxiety. *Check plasma sodium level in patients taking antidepressants if not checked recently.*
Antiepileptic drugs	Antiepileptic drugs can cause sedation, falls, confusion, and paradoxical disinhibition. Valproate may cause hyperammonemia. Levetiracetam may cause psychiatric symptoms. *In patients taking valproate, check ammonia level.*
Antihypertensives	β-Blockers may be associated with fatigue and depression. Diuretics can cause hyponatremia.
Antiparkinsonian agents	Levodopa and dopamine receptor agonists can cause hallucinations, compulsions, and fatigue. Anticholinergic agents (e.g., benztropine) have the same problems as those listed above.
Antipsychotics	Antipsychotics can cause akathisia, which may manifest as restlessness, wandering, or physical aggression.

TABLE 4–4. Medications and other substances that can cause behavioral and psychological symptoms of dementia (BPSD) (*continued*)

Medications or substance	Comments and recommendations
Cannabis	Cannabis may cause anxiety, paranoia, and apathy. Cannabis use is likely to become more prevalent among older adults. *Consider urine drug toxicology.*
Cholinesterase inhibitors	Cholinesterase inhibitors can cause insomnia, nightmares, loss of appetite, and weight loss.
Complementary and alternative medicine approaches	St. John's wort taken in combination with an SSRI or SNRI could cause serotonin syndrome, which may manifest as anxiety, restlessness, wandering, or physical aggression. Complementary and alternative interventions are not well studied in older adults.
Opioids	Either use or withdrawal of opioids may be associated with BPSD, falls, and cognitive impairment.
Sedative-hypnotic medications	Either use or withdrawal of sedative-hypnotic medications may be associated with BPSD, falls, and cognitive impairment. Benzodiazepines can cause paradoxical disinhibition; "z-drugs" can cause nighttime behavioral disturbance.
Steroids	Steroids may be associated with a wide range of symptoms, including depression, anxiety, aggression, and psychosis.
Supplements	Excess use of calcium supplements could result in hypercalcemia.

Note.   SNRI=serotonin-norepinephrine reuptake inhibitor; SSRI=selective serotonin reuptake inhibitor.

pose. Although these capacities deteriorate over time, they are important factors in understanding why a person is experiencing BPSD.

A number of psychological threats are particularly relevant to people with dementia. Grief and loss are nearly universal experiences as one ages. Patients with dementia may have a difficult time with bereavement; a particularly nightmarish scenario is when a person repeatedly forgets that a loved one has died and then experiences the loss anew each time he or she is reminded. Boredom is very common, especially in institutional settings that offer limited opportunities for cognitive stimulation and social engagement; depression and anxiety may lead to withdrawal from activities, which then exacerbates boredom. Patients with dementia may cite embarrassment about perceived and actual cognitive and physical impairments as a reason for avoiding or withdrawing from social engagements. Some patients with dementia may feel that they are a burden on their family members, which in turn may contribute to guilt, depression, or suicidal ideation. Unfortunately, as patients become increasingly dependent on others for help with activities of daily living—especially dressing and bathing—loss of dignity can become a real concern. Suicidal ideation can arise, and patients with dementia may be at higher risk of suicide. Finally, loss of control and autonomy can threaten one's identity, self-worth, and integrity.

Patients' premorbid personality traits may help predict how they will respond to the stressors of dementia. (I tell caregivers that patients do not "check their personalities at the door" of the assisted living facility or nursing home.) As discussed in the section "Etiological Models of BPSD" in Chapter 3, the most consistent finding in the literature is that premorbid neuroticism (proneness to emotional arousal and negativity) is associated with mood disturbance and aggression. In addition, premorbid Cluster A (solitary or paranoid) personality structure is associated with anxiety, depression, and hallucinations, whereas Cluster C (avoidant or dependent) personality structure is associated with depression (Prior et al. 2016). Other anecdotal observations: Patients with obsessive-compulsive personality traits (e.g., being rigid, rule bound, and excessively goal oriented) may find excessive fault in the care they are receiving and as a result become irritable or aggressive; their perceiving caregivers' responses as inadequate no matter what the caregivers do may lead to caregiver burnout. Patients with narcissistic personality traits may become angry or aggressive if they find that others are not paying sufficient attention to them; they may also become depressed and withdrawn in the face of cognitive and functional decline, which they may perceive as humiliating (so-called narcissistic injury).

The lifetime prevalence of trauma in the general population of adults is estimated to be 70%–90% (Ganzel 2018), yet most people do not develop posttraumatic stress disorder (PTSD). Those older adults who do have a history of PTSD are at increased risk of developing dementia (Yaffe et al. 2010). Furthermore, the development of dementia renders the individual less able to control symptoms of PTSD and biologically more vulnerable to recurrence of the disorder. Screening for a history of trauma (childhood abuse, sexual assault, domestic violence, exposure to combat, surviving the

Holocaust or other wartime experiences, and current elder abuse) and PTSD is an important part of understanding potential comorbid conditions that may exacerbate BPSD and complicate the response to BPSD (Reus et al. 2016).

Patients with dementia may have preexisting psychiatric conditions other than PTSD. Depression, bipolar disorder, schizophrenia, anxiety disorder, and alcohol use disorder are all associated with higher risk of developing dementia (Zilkens et al. 2014), so it stands to reason that patients with a history of these conditions are overrepresented among patients with dementia. Diagnostic confusion may result because it may not be clear if psychiatric symptoms should be attributed to dementia (and labeled BPSD) or viewed as a recurrence of a psychiatric disorder. For example, in a patient with bipolar disorder who later develops AD, it may be unclear if an episode of aggression or psychosis is due to bipolar disorder and should be treated accordingly (i.e., with lithium, anticonvulsants, or antipsychotics) or requires the management of BPSD, as described in Chapter 5.

As discussed in Chapter 3, the unmet needs model can be particularly helpful in understanding the psychological contributions to BPSD. For example, unmet psychological needs—for dignity, autonomy, sense of purpose and meaning, feeling loved and appreciated, and intimacy—may contribute to a wide range of BPSD, including depression, anxiety, restlessness, verbal or physical aggression, and inappropriate sexual behaviors.

As dementia progresses, the patient's capacity for making decisions about his or her medical and personal care diminishes. Although assessment of decisional capacity is not immediately required as part of the assessment of BPSD, it may become necessary in order to determine a patient's ability to consent to treatment of BPSD. I discuss the assessment of decisional capacity in detail in the section "Decisional Capacity and Other Capacities" in Chapter 7.

In summary, a comprehensive assessment of the patient's premorbid psychological functioning may not be feasible immediately after BPSD become a concern but should be undertaken at some point. The process could begin with an open-ended question to family members, such as "What was the patient like before dementia?" Additional history would then be obtained regarding the patient's "likes and dislikes, lifestyle, hobbies, intimacy and relationship patterns" (Reus et al. 2016, p. 14). The patient can be interviewed to determine how he or she "interpret[s] the meaning of and navigate[s] the difficult terrain associated with dementia and its symptoms" (Reus et al. 2016, p. 14). Finally, it should be noted that premorbid personality structure may in fact be a source of resilience and the ability to cope with stress—that is, a protective or mitigating factor in the expression of BPSD. Building on a patient's strengths may be as or more productive than focusing only on deficits.

PSYCHOSOCIAL AND ENVIRONMENTAL FACTORS

Humans perform best when exposed to optimal levels of stress: too much stress can result in anxiety, irritability, withdrawal, avoidance, fight-or-flight responses, and decreased cognition and functioning; too little stress can result in boredom and inactivity. The progressively lowered stress threshold model, described in Chapter 3, ascribes BPSD to a mismatch between the level of stress and the ability of the person with dementia to respond appropriately to stress, which declines over the course of dementia (Smith et al. 2004). Psychosocial stressors that are particularly relevant to persons with dementia and other older adults include the following:

- *Interpersonal stressors:* Patients with dementia often experience strain in their relationships with family members and with other caregivers. Long-standing interpersonal dysfunction, such as problems with communication, may become especially apparent when one or both members of the dyad develop(s) dementia. Separation from family members (e.g., children and grandchildren living in different cities) can be challenging. Illness in family members can result in worry about those family members; patients with dementia may in fact be or have been caregivers for their spouses or partners. The most severe interpersonal stressor, of course, is death of a spouse or partner.
- *Financial stressors:* Many older adults have fixed incomes and may face rising costs associated with food, housing, and health care. In early-onset dementia, the patient may still be working; continued work may itself be a stressor, and worry about losing one's job and associated financial and psychological implications may arise. Access to health care may be compromised. Food insecurity may become a problem, especially for older adults living alone or with low income.
- *Safety concerns and violence:* Caregivers may be neglectful, emotionally abusive, physically abusive, sexually abusive, or financially exploitative. Patient concerns about cooking, driving, taking medications correctly, and falling may also be stressors. Patients with dementia may live alone or in unsafe neighborhoods, leading to anxiety and perhaps even what clinicians could construe as paranoia.

BPSD arise in the context of the environment in which the person with dementia is living. Among the many benefits of staying in one's own home are the familiarity of objects and activities, experiencing a sense of belonging, and viewing the home as place for retreat, rejuvenation, safety, and security—presumably all protective factors (Førsund et al. 2018). However, a number of factors at home could contribute to BPSD and other safety concerns; these factors include clutter (e.g., stacks of newspapers or boxes), access to sharp objects, poor lighting, and lack of cognitive and social activities (Marquardt et al. 2011; Struckmeyer and Pickens 2016). Transitions in residence can be particularly challenging for patients with dementia, especially moves from home to a long-term care setting but also moves to a hospital or subacute rehabilitation facility (Førsund et al. 2018). Factors within long-term care that might contribute to BPSD include ambient noise, busyness of the environment, problems with lighting, uncomfortable room temperature, institutional (as opposed to homelike and personalized) ambience, rules and restrictions, homesickness, lack of privacy, and monotony (Førsund et al. 2018; Marquardt et al. 2014).

CULTURAL AND SPIRITUAL FACTORS

Culture refers to a "a set of shared symbols, beliefs and customs that shapes individual and/or group behavior" (Dilworth-Anderson and Gibson 2002, p. S56). Cultural factors may affect how patients and family members interpret the symptoms of dementia, may determine whether or not medical attention is sought, and may interfere with access to health care (e.g., because of language barriers) (Mukadam et al. 2011). For example, ethnic minority elders and their family members may view dementia as a normal part of aging and not a medical process. A common theme across multiple ethnic groups is the role of "pressure" (or stress or worry) in the pathogenesis of dementia—that is, excess anxiety throughout one's life leads to dementia (Dilworth-Anderson and Gibson 2002). The prevalence of many BPSD is similar among Mexican Americans, African Americans, and non-Hispanic whites in the United States, except that apathy and delusions appear to be less common among Mexican Americans (Salazar et al. 2015). Cultural expectations around the responsibilities of children and grandchildren with respect to the elders may affect the relationships among patients and family caregivers (Dilworth-Anderson and Gibson 2002).

The American Psychiatric Association's Cultural Formulation Interview (CFI) may help enhance clinicians' understanding of the role of a patient's culture in BPSD (Lewis-Fernández et al. 2015). The Informant Version of the CFI instructs the interviewer to tell the informant (family member or other caregiver): "Sometimes, aspects of people's background or identity can make the [problem] better or worse. By *background* or *identity*, I mean, for example, the communities you belong to, the languages you speak, where you or your family are from, your race or ethnic background, your gender or sexual orientation, and your faith or religion" (p. 296). The interviewer then asks the informant what the most important aspects of the patient's background or identity are; whether there are any aspects of the patient's background or identity that makes a difference to the presenting problem; and whether there are any aspects of the patient's background or identity that are causing other concerns or difficulties. The interviewer also notes that "sometimes doctors and patients misunderstand each other because they come from different backgrounds" (p. 297) and then asks if the informant has been concerned about this and how it can be addressed. The full version of the CFI–Informant Version is available online (www.psychiatry.org/ File%20Library/Psychiatrists/Practice/DSM/APA_DSM5_Cultural-Formulation-Interview-Informant.pdf). The following describes a case in which cultural considerations are particularly relevant.

Case Example 4–1: "Mom Doesn't Want to Do Anything Anymore."

Mrs. Phan is a 68-year-old Cambodian woman with vascular dementia who lives at home with her husband and youngest daughter. She has a history of PTSD related to her imprisonment in a work camp during the despotic Khmer Rouge regime; she and her family escaped to the United States in the early 1980s. She had been treated with paroxetine with some relief of symptoms of PTSD, but recently her family has noted more emotional problems. They report that over the past year or so, she has withdrawn from many activities, including family get-togethers, going to Buddhist temple, and playing the flute (a passion of hers since childhood). Mrs. Phan's husband and daughter chide her frequently and have found themselves very frustrated because she has spent more and more time in her room, watching television or sleeping during the daytime. Her daughter, Kolab, brings Mrs. Phan to her doctor, seeking a treatment to make her more active and interested again. Her family does not have any concerns about her or their safety.

The doctor schedules a 40-minute office visit to complete a comprehensive evaluation with an interpreter present. The chief concern appears to be either apathy or depression or both. Mrs. Phan denies feeling sad; Kolab does not recall her mother crying or expressing hopelessness or suicidal ideation. Mrs. Phan's lack of interest has been present for the past year, does not have any obvious precipitants, is present throughout the day, and has resulted in her friends and extended family visiting her less often. Kolab admits that she and her father respond by berating Mrs. Phan, who then withdraws further.

The doctor screens for other BPSD and finds that Mrs. Phan has been sleeping poorly (with many nightmares), has been fearful that someone will enter her home and abduct her family members (as happened when she lived in Cambodia), and has had periodic visual hallucinations of strangers within her home. Because she has been sleeping poorly, her family recently bought her an OTC sleep agent containing diphenhydramine, which she takes two or three times per night without benefit. In addition to paroxetine for PTSD, her medications include hydrochlorothiazide for hypertension, cyclobenzaprine for chronic low back pain, metformin for diabetes mellitus type 2, and cetirizine for allergic rhinitis. Mrs. Phan does not drink alcohol, smoke tobacco, or use any illicit drugs. Kolab admits that she and her father have been under a fair amount of stress but denies that they themselves are depressed.

With Kolab out of the examination room, the doctor screens for elder abuse but does not find any evidence. A physical examination is unremarkable, except that the patient winces in pain when her back is examined, and she in general sits uncomfortably in her chair; her vital signs are normal; her body mass index is elevated at 31 kg/m². She is alert and oriented to place and time, though her memory for recent events is poor. Her affect is sullen, but she denies any suicidal ideation. She denies auditory hallucinations but endorses visual hallucinations and paranoia, as described. She is easily fatigued and sleeps during the day.

Mrs. Phan has not had any recent laboratory tests done. The most recent neuroimaging was a magnetic resonance imaging (MRI) scan of the brain 2 years earlier that helped confirm the diagnosis of vascular dementia, with extensive confluent ischemic disease throughout deep white matter areas of the brain.

Mrs. Phan's doctor suspects that she has apathy, paranoia, and visual hallucinations associated with vascular dementia, as well as a recurrence of PTSD. A basic metabolic panel is ordered to rule out hyponatremia, because Mrs. Phan is taking a selective serotonin reuptake inhibitor and a thiazide diuretic, and to rule out dehydration, given her withdrawal from activities. A thyroid-stimulating hormone test is ordered to rule out hypothyroidism. Polysomnography is ordered to rule obstructive sleep apnea. Mrs. Phan's doctor recommends discontinuation of diphenhydramine because of its anticholinergic effect and suggests that she switch to another antidepressant because paroxetine is also anticholinergic. The doctor wonders if her recent estrangement from family and friends and lack of participation in spiritual activities are both consequences of and contributors to apathy. The doctor suggests that Kolab and her father attend caregiver support groups to learn how to more effectively respond to Mrs. Phan's withdrawal from activities.

Just as persons with dementia remain psychological beings, they also remain spiritual beings, though perhaps less able to express their spiritual needs over time. Religious beliefs and practices may inform how patients react to the diagnosis of dementia and how they cope with dementia (Beuscher and Beck 2008). Religious practices such as prayer and attending religious services may foster optimism, resilience, and serenity and may promote engagement and a sense of belonging to a community—that is, they may serve as protective factors with respect to BPSD (Ødbehr et al. 2017).

ROLE OF THE FAMILY AND OTHER CAREGIVERS

A critical component of assessing BPSD is determining how family members and other caregivers understand and respond to BPSD and how they interact with the patient (Kales et al. 2014). Caregivers may unwittingly cause or exacerbate symptoms by asking cognitively challenging questions; rushing the patient in carrying out tasks; or expressing their own anger, anxiety, or depression (Reus et al. 2016). Caregivers may interpret patients' behaviors as volitional and perhaps even manipulative, caregivers' expectations about the patients' cognitive and functional abilities may be inaccurate, and caregivers may underreport symptoms due to a wish not to "air dirty laundry" to outsiders (Kales et al. 2014).

As discussed in the section "Effects of BPSD on Patients, Caregivers, and Society" in Chapter 3, caregivers themselves may have clinically significant depression or anxiety. My own practice is to screen for depression in family caregivers with the PHQ-2 (Löwe et al. 2005): "Over the last 2 weeks, have you felt down, depressed, or hopeless? Have you had little interest or pleasure in doing things?" Answering "yes" to either question is not diagnostic of depression but suggests that further evaluation of the caregiver, for example by his or her primary care provider, should take place (Maurer 2012). Finally, as discussed in Chapter 2 (see the section "Screening for Elder Abuse" and Table 2–3), the clinician should screen for elder abuse.

SUMMARY: ASSESSING A PERSON WITH BPSD

The primary goal of assessing BPSD is collecting the information necessary to develop an understanding of why BPSD have arisen, with a view to developing a treatment plan. If the safety of the patient or those around the patient is at risk, then the initial assessment may need to be abbreviated. The following describes the case of a patient with imminent safety concerns.

Case Example 4–2: "He's Going to Hurt Someone Badly—You Need to Do Something Now!"

Mr. Abdullah is a 57-year-old married computer engineer who was diagnosed with FTD 2 years ago. He was initially thought to have bipolar disorder on account of his impulsivity and mood swings, but cognitive decline and progressive problems at work led his primary care provider to suspect dementia. An MRI of the brain revealed atrophy of the frontal lobes and anterior horns of the temporal lobes bilaterally, consistent with a diagnosis of FTD.

One month ago, his wife and children decided that he should move into an assisted living facility. He had stopped working a year earlier, was no longer able to drive, and required constant supervision at home due to wandering. His family felt that they could no longer safely care for him at home, and he grudgingly agreed to move to a higher level of care.

Mr. Abdullah has been living at Pleasant Gardens Memory Care Unit for the past week, and it has not gone well. Each day, the nursing director of the facility has called his wife and his primary care physician to report escalating problems with behavior—specifically, his angry refusals of assistance with activities of daily living. In the most recent incident, Mr. Abdullah fled from staff when they attempted to bathe him and then tried to kick and punch them when they cornered him. On one occasion, he grabbed and twisted the arm of a certified nursing assistant, and she was unable to complete her shift. He has been telling his family that he wants to return home because "everyone here is 20 years older than me" and he does not feel that he belongs at the facility; formerly a daily jogger, he feels confined on the unit. The director of nursing informs the primary care physician that something must be done to curtail Mr. Abdullah's behavior; if not, Pleasant Gardens may no longer be able to care for him.

Given the seriousness of the situation, the physician conducts an abbreviated assessment of Mr. Abdullah's BPSD. The chief symptom of concern is physical aggression toward the staff, which occurs every time a staff member offers him assistance. The behaviors can happen any time of day but are worst around dinnertime, when there is a fair amount of activity at Pleasant Gardens. His vital signs have been normal. He has been up at night a fair amount with nocturia but otherwise has no new physical symptoms. The physician notes that Mr. Abdullah recently (within the past month) had a complete set of labs prior to admission to the facility. Mr. Abdullah has a history of recurrent UTIs, and his wife says that his nocturia seems to have been worse over the past week. The physician reviews the medication list, which includes atenolol for hypertension, atorvastatin for dyslipidemia, and low-dose aspirin to reduce risk of myocardial infarction, all of which he has taken for years; there are no new medications. Mr. Abdullah does not drink alcohol, and the physician does not suspect illicit drug use.

The primary care physician's initial impression is that Mr. Abdullah's physical aggression represents an exacerbation of behavioral symptoms associated with FTD, likely due to his move out of his home and into a novel environment. His index of suspicion for medical etiology is low, except for a UTI, so he orders a urinalysis. The physician develops a plan to have family present once daily at dinnertime, when staff will also assist him with activities of daily living; the physician asks the facility to designate one staff member as the primary caregiver so as to reduce the number of transitions and unfamiliar faces for Mr. Abdullah; the facility arranges for twice-daily off-unit physical exercise for Mr. Abdullah with a staff member who is referred to as his "exercise buddy"; and the physician and the nursing director arrange for the staff to immediately receive additional training on the care of patients with FTD.

Ultimately, prior to developing a plan to help a patient with BPSD, all of the following steps should take place: fully describing the primary symptom; screening for other BPSD; evaluating medical etiologies and ruling out delirium; reviewing the medication list (and other substances used) for potential offenders; appreciating psychological factors such as loneliness, boredom, and fear; identifying psychosocial, environmental, cultural, and spiritual factors that might be predisposing, precipitating, or protective factors; assessing caregivers and how they respond to BPSD; and screening for elder abuse. Figure 4–5 provides a summary, including pathways for when safety is and is not a concern.

KEY POINTS

- An important step in understanding and addressing BPSD is diagnosing the cause of mild or major neurocognitive disorder. In a crisis precipitated by BPSD, this may not be immediately feasible, but establishing the correct underlying diagnosis should eventually occur.

- Each behavioral or psychological symptom of concern should be fully ascertained with respect to timing, severity, antecedents, consequences, and whether or not it is new or different. Although there may a specific behavioral or psychological symptom of concern, clinicians should screen for other BPSD.

- Clinicians and facilities should consider employing a structured, evidence-based framework for assessing BPSD, such as the Targeted Interdisciplinary Model for Evaluation and Treatment of Neuropsychiatric Symptoms (TIME). Other frameworks to consider include "describe, investigate, create, evaluate" (DICE) and the Wisconsin Star Method.

- Rating scales may be useful in assessing the presence and severity of BPSD as well as the patient's response to interventions. A variety of rating scales may cover BPSD broadly or may cover specific BPSD (e.g., depression, anxiety).

- Clinicians should consider the possibility of medical (metabolic, infectious, central nervous system, and other) etiologies and conduct the requisite evaluation.

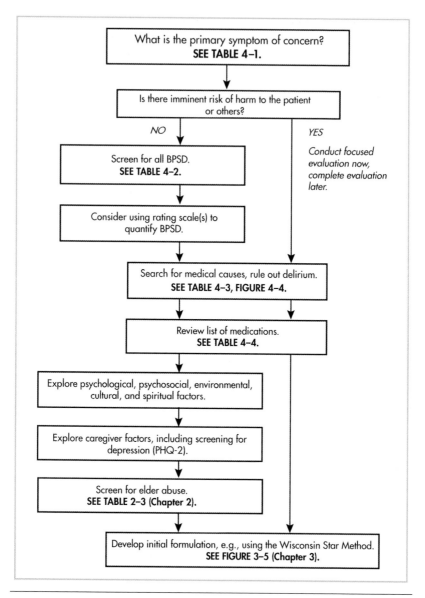

FIGURE 4–5. Summary of assessing behavioral and psychological symptoms of dementia (BPSD).

PHQ-2 = Patient Health Questionnaire–2 (see text).

- Clinicians should carefully scrutinize the medication list, looking closely at any recent additions or changes and bearing in mind that patients may take OTC medications and supplements in addition to prescribed medications. Use of alcohol, cannabis, and illicit substances should also be assessed.

- Psychological factors that could contribute to BPSD (and that could be targets of intervention) include boredom, loneliness, grief, fear, embarrassment, loss of control or autonomy, loss of dignity, and feeling like one is a burden.

  - Premorbid personality traits can influence the expression of BPSD.

  - A history of trauma is not uncommon in people with dementia, suggesting that trauma-informed care may be especially relevant.

  - Preexisting psychiatric disorders are not uncommon in patients with dementia and can confound the presentation of BPSD.

- Clinicians also should screen for caregiver factors, including how caregivers respond to BPSD, caregivers' own depression or anxiety, and potential elder abuse.

- Interpersonal stressors, financial stressors, safety concerns, environmental factors, cultural background, and spirituality may all contribute to or mitigate BPSD and should be assessed.

RESOURCES FOR PATIENTS, FAMILIES, AND CAREGIVERS

Family Caregiver Alliance: Dementia, Caregiving, and Controlling Frustration. San Francisco, CA, Family Caregiver Alliance, 2003. Available at: https://www.caregiver.org/dementia-caregiving-and-controlling-frustration. This web page is directed toward helping caregivers appreciate the stresses of caregiving and recognize the warning signs of frustration.

Family Caregiver Alliance: Alzheimer's Disease and Caregiving. San Francisco, CA, Family Caregiver Alliance, 2012. Available at: https://www.caregiver.org/alzheimers-disease-caregiving. This web page comprehensively explains what caregivers can expect in AD by stage of illness.

Frontotemporal Dementia Caregiver Support Center: Caregiver Issues—Managing Behaviors, 2006. Available at: http://www.ftdsupport.com/cgi-behaviors.htm. This web page very nicely presents the ABCs (Antecedent, Behavior, Consequences) approach to describing behavioral and psychological symptoms of dementia and explains how this approach can be used to develop a treatment plan.

National Institute on Aging: Communication and Behavior Problems: Resources for Alzheimer's Caregivers. Bethesda, MD, National Institute on Aging, 2017. Available at: https://www.nia.nih.gov/health/communication-and-behavior-problems-resources-alzheimers-caregivers. This web page lists a variety of resources related to understanding BPSD. Topics include common changes in personality and behavior, other factors that can affect behavior, and tips for caregivers.

Steinman MA, Fick DM: Using wisely: a reminder on the proper use of the American Geriatrics Society Beers Criteria. J Am Geriatr Soc 67(4):644–646, 2019. Available at: https://www.ncbi.nlm.nih.gov/pmc/articles/PMC5325682. The authors of this paper, which is available via open access, aim to explain to patients and clinicians the intended role of the Beers Criteria for potentially inappropriate medication use. They argue that the criteria should serve as a "starting point for a comprehensive process of identifying and improving medication appropriateness and safety."

REFERENCES

Ahmed A, van der Marck MA, van den Elsen G, et al: Cannabinoids in late-onset Alzheimer's disease. Clin Pharmacol Ther 97(6):597–606, 2015 25788394

Alexopoulos GS, Abrams RC, Young RC, et al: Cornell Scale for Depression in Dementia. Biol Psychiatry 23(3):271–284, 1988 3337862

American Geriatrics Society 2019 Beers Criteria Update Expert Panel: American Geriatrics Society 2019 updated Beers Criteria for Potentially Inappropriate Medication Use in Older Adults. J Am Geriatr Soc 67(4):674–694, 2019 30693946

American Psychiatric Association: Diagnostic and Statistical Manual of Mental Disorders, 5th Edition. Arlington, VA, American Psychiatric Association, 2013

Arcury TA, Grzywacz JG, Neiberg RH, et al: Older adults' self-management of daily symptoms: complementary therapies, self-care, and medical care. J Aging Health 24(4):569–597, 2012 22187091

Arcury TA, Nguyen HT, Sandberg JC, et al: Use of complementary therapies for health promotion among older adults. J Appl Gerontol 34(5):552–572, 2015 24652893

Beuscher L, Beck C: A literature review of spirituality in coping with early stage Alzheimer's disease. J Clin Nurs 17(5A):88–97, 2008 18298759

Cohen-Mansfield J: Agitated behaviors in the elderly, II: preliminary results in the cognitively deteriorated. J Am Geriatr Soc 34(10):722–727, 1986 3760436

D'Agata E, Loeb MB, Mitchell SL: Challenges in assessing nursing home residents with advanced dementia for suspected urinary tract infections. J Am Geriatr Soc 61(1):62–66, 2013 23311553

Dilworth-Anderson P, Gibson BE: The cultural influence of values, norms, meanings, and perceptions in understanding dementia in ethnic minorities. Alzheimer Dis Assoc Disord 16 (suppl 2):S56–S63, 2002 12351916

Førsund LH, Grov EK, Helvik A-S, et al: The experience of lived space in persons with dementia: a systematic meta-synthesis. BMC Geriatr 18(1):33, 2018 29390970

Ganzel BL: Trauma-informed hospice and palliative care. Gerontologist 58(3):409–419, 2018 27927732

Han BH, Moore AA: Prevention and screening of unhealthy substance use by older adults. Clin Geriatr Med 34(1):117–129, 2018 29129212

Hölttä E, Laakkonen M-L, Laurila JV, et al: The overlap of delirium with neuropsychiatric symptoms among patients with dementia. Am J Geriatr Psychiatry 19(12):1034–1041, 2011 22123275

Inouye SK, van Dyck CH, Alessi CA, et al: Clarifying confusion: the Confusion Assessment Method. A new method for detection of delirium. Ann Intern Med 113(12):941–948, 1990 2240918

Jump RLP, Crnich CJ, Mody L, et al: Infectious diseases in older adults of long-term care facilities: update on approach to diagnosis and management. J Am Geriatr Soc 66(4):789–803, 2018 29667186

Kales HC, Gitlin LN, Lyketsos CG: Management of neuropsychiatric symptoms of dementia in clinical settings: recommendations from a multidisciplinary expert panel. J Am Geriatr Soc 62(4):762–769, 2014 24635665

Kaufer DI, Cummings JL, Ketchel P, et al: Validation of the NPI-Q, a brief clinical form of the Neuropsychiatric Inventory. J Neuropsychiatry Clin Neurosci 12(2):233–239, 2000 11001602

Lewis-Fernández R: Aggarwal NK, Hinton L, et al: DSM-5 Handbook on the Cultural Formulation Interview. Arlington, VA, American Psychiatric Association, 2015

Lichtwarck B, Tvera A-M, Roen I: Targeted Interdisciplinary Model for Evaluation and Treatment of Neuropsychiatric Symptoms—Manual, 2nd Edition. Ottestad, Norway, Centre for Old Age Psychiatric Research, Innlandet Hospital Trust, 2017

Lichtwarck B, Selbaek G, Kirkevold Ø, et al: Targeted interdisciplinary model for evaluation and treatment of neuropsychiatric symptoms: a cluster randomized controlled trial. Am J Geriatr Psychiatry 26(1):25–38, 2018 28669575

Löwe B, Kroenke K, Gräfe K: Detecting and monitoring depression with a two-item questionnaire (PHQ-2). J Psychosom Res 58(2):163–171 2005 15820844

Marquardt G, Johnston D, Black BS, et al: A descriptive study of home modifications for people with dementia and barriers to implementation. J Hous Elder 25(3):258–273, 2011 21904419

Marquardt G, Bueter K, Motzek T: Impact of the design of the built environment on people with dementia: an evidence-based review. HERD 8(1):127–157, 2014 25816188

Maurer DM: Screening for depression. Am Fam Physician 85(2):139–144, 2012 22335214

Mukadam N, Cooper C, Livingston G: A systematic review of ethnicity and pathways to care in dementia. Int J Geriatr Psychiatry 26(1):12–20, 2011 21157846

Ødbehr LS, Hauge S, Danbolt LJ, et al: Residents' and caregivers' views on spiritual care and their understanding of spiritual needs in persons with dementia: a meta-synthesis. Dementia 16(7):911–929, 2017 26721285

Prior J, Abraham R, Nicholas H, et al: Are premorbid abnormal personality traits associated with behavioural and psychological symptoms in dementia? Int J Geriatr Psychiatry 31(9):1050–1055, 2016 26968137

Reisberg B, Borenstein J, Salob SP, et al: Behavioral symptoms in Alzheimer's disease: phenomenology and treatment. J Clin Psychiatry 48 (suppl):9–15, 1987 3553166

Reus VI, Fochtmann LJ, Eyler AE, et al: The American Psychiatric Association practice guideline on the use of antipsychotics to treat agitation or psychosis in patients with dementia. Am J Psychiatry 173(5):543–546, 2016 27133416

Salazar R, Royall DR, Palmer RF: Neuropsychiatric symptoms in community-dwelling Mexican-Americans: results from the Hispanic Established Population for Epidemiological Study of the Elderly (HEPESE) study. Int J Geriatr Psychiatry 30(3):300–307, 2015 24838594

Shankar KK, Walker M, Frost D, et al: The development of a valid and reliable scale for rating anxiety in dementia (RAID). Aging Ment Health 3(1):39–49, 1999

Smith M, Gerdner LA, Hall GR, et al: History, development, and future of the progressively lowered stress threshold: a conceptual model for dementia care. J Am Geriatr Soc 52(10):1755–1760, 2004 15450057

Struckmeyer LR, Pickens ND: Home modifications for people with Alzheimer's disease: a scoping review. Am J Occup Ther 70(1):1–9, 2016 26709430

van Buul LW, Vreeken HL, Bradley SF, et al: The development of a decision tool for the empiric treatment of suspected urinary tract infection in frail older adults: a Delphi consensus procedure. J Am Med Dir Assoc 19(9):757–764, 2018 29910137

Wood S, Cummings JL, Hsu MA, et al: The use of the Neuropsychiatric Inventory in nursing home residents: characterization and measurement. Am J Geriatr Psychiatry 8(1):75–83, 2000 10648298

Yaffe K, Vittinghoff E, Lindquist K, et al: Posttraumatic stress disorder and risk of dementia among U.S. veterans. Arch Gen Psychiatry 67(6):608–613, 2010 20530010

Zilkens RR, Bruce DG, Duke J, et al: Severe psychiatric disorders in mid-life and risk of dementia in late-life (age 65–84 years): a population based case-control study. Curr Alzheimer Res 11(7):681–693, 2014 25115541

CHAPTER 5

MANAGEMENT OF BEHAVIORAL AND PSYCHOLOGICAL SYMPTOMS OF DEMENTIA

Précis

The assessment of a patient with behavioral and psychological symptoms of dementia (BPSD) informs the treatment approach. Any medical problems, environmental factors, or medications that are determined to be contributing to the symptoms should be addressed. It is essential to train, educate, and support caregivers—in fact, caregiver training is among the most clearly effective interventions for BPSD. Other approaches that may be of benefit include increasing a patient's level of activity, providing adequate cognitive and sensory stimulation, music therapy, and behavioral management. Interventions should be culturally sensitive and tailored to the needs of patients and their caregivers. Pharmacological interventions can also be effective but should be used only if nonpharmacological approaches have been ineffective or if a patient's behaviors are markedly distressing to the patient or dangerous to the patient or to others. The medications with the strongest evidence for efficacy are antipsychotics—but they can have serious side effects, including an increased risk of mortality. Antidepressants are likely safer than antipsychotics but are less clearly effective. Adequately addressing pain, even with an intervention as straightforward as scheduling acetaminophen, can be very helpful. Other pharmacological options include cognitive enhancers, prazosin, dextromethorphan-quinidine, carbamazepine, methylphenidate, and, in limited circumstances, benzodiazepines and pimavanserin. Clinicians must carefully monitor for side effects and should strongly consider eventual discontinuation of psychotropic medications. Most of the literature on treating BPSD applies to patients with

131

dementia due to Alzheimer's disease (AD); there are special considerations for using medications in treating patients with vascular dementia, dementia with Lewy bodies (DLB), frontotemporal dementia (FTD), and dementia due to intellectual or developmental disability.

OVERVIEW OF MANAGEMENT STRATEGY

Effective treatment of BPSD requires an understanding of patients, their caregivers, and their environment. One of the goals of the assessment of BPSD, as described in Chapter 4, is to identify medical, environmental, and psychosocial problems that could be precipitating or perpetuating BPSD (Rabins et al. 2007). The clinician should address any potential medical contributions and discontinue potentially offending medications or substances, as discussed further in the next section, "Addressing Medical and Medication/Substance–Related Causes." In general, I recommend against adding new medications—rather, the focus of treatment should be on nonpharmacological interventions for patients and their caregivers.

Caring for patients with dementia is a skill that must be acquired, and it is also an emotionally taxing experience. Among the interventions for BPSD with the clearest efficacy is training family and staff in the care of patients with dementia (Kales et al. 2015). This includes education regarding the nature of dementia and BPSD, training in how to assess BPSD, and training in using behavioral and environmental interventions. Support and respite for caregivers, including monitoring for caregiver depression and anxiety, are also critical (Rabins et al. 2007). I cover caregiver interventions in further detail in the section "Support and Education of Family and Other Caregivers."

A wide range of nonpharmacological interventions may address BPSD, though the evidence for efficacy is somewhat mixed (Livingston et al. 2014). A behavioral approach identifies BPSD antecedents or precipitants that could be avoided or mitigated; views the responses of family members and other caregivers as capable of influencing behaviors, either positively or negatively; and implements responses to behaviors that will hopefully reduce the frequency and severity of those behaviors. Other elements of a behavioral management plan might include increasing cognitive and sensory stimulation for patients, modifying their environment, music therapy, adequate light exposure, and exercise. Individual psychotherapy may be effective for patients with less severe cognitive impairment (Orgeta et al. 2015). Manualized approaches such as the Targeted Interdisciplinary Model for Evaluation and Treatment of Neuropsychiatric Symptoms (TIME; Lichtwarck et al. 2018) and "describe, investigate, create, evaluate" (DICE; Kales et al. 2014), both introduced in Chapter 4, may help provide family members and other caregivers with a framework for understanding and managing behaviors. I discuss nonpharmacological approaches in greater detail below, in the section "Nonpharmacological Interventions."

If behavioral measures have failed, if the patient is experiencing significant distress, or if behaviors pose a threat to the patient or others, a psychopharmacological intervention may be warranted. There are several caveats:

1. Patients with dementia often may already be coping with significant polypharmacy, which may in and of itself contribute to cognitive impairment and BPSD (Rongen et al. 2016).
2. Clinical trials have generally shown that medications are only modestly effective for BPSD (Wang et al. 2015).
3. There are significant risks associated with the use of medications for BPSD, especially the risk of mortality with antipsychotics (Reus et al. 2016).
4. In North America, there are no medications approved by regulatory agencies for treatment of BPSD; in Europe, only risperidone is approved (Porsteinsson and Antonsdottir 2017).

If the decision is made to prescribe a medication, I generally recommend starting with an antidepressant and reserving antipsychotics for when there is very significant distress or danger. Medications are typically started at lower dosages and titrated more slowly in older adults than in younger adults. Obtaining informed consent may be a challenge because patients themselves may not have the capacity to consent to a medication (Walaszek 2011). Once a medication is started, the clinician must monitor the outcome and consider eventually discontinuing the medication (Reus et al. 2016). The section "Pharmacological Interventions" later in this chapter reviews medications in detail.

Table 5–1 summarizes how to address BPSD. These suggestions presuppose, however, that a patient's behavior does not pose an immediate risk to self or others, including caregivers, other household members (e.g., a frail partner, grandchildren), and other residents in a long-term care (LTC) facility—in other words, a safe setting and adequate time are needed to methodically follow the steps listed in Table 5–1. Otherwise, the patient may need to be evaluated and treated in a safer and more highly monitored setting, such as an emergency department or inpatient medical or psychiatric unit (Rabins et al. 2007). The decision to treat the patient in a different set-

---

TABLE 5–1.   Summary of how to address behavioral and psychological
symptoms of dementia

---

1. Treat underlying medical causes.

2. Discontinue offending medications and substances.

3. Support and educate caregivers and other family members.

4. Develop a psychological/behavioral/environmental management plan—see Table 5–4.

5. Avoid adding new medications, unless there is risk of harm to patient or others.

6. If a pharmacological strategy is chosen, select one of the following:

   a.   Antidepressants—see Table 5–5

   b.   Antipsychotics—see Table 5–6

   c.   Other pharmacological approaches—see Table 5–7

7. If a medication is added, regularly monitor outcomes and attempt discontinuation.

8. Ensure that patients and caregivers are in a safe environment.

---

ting brings its own challenges, however, in that moving a patient to a novel environment with unfamiliar staff may exacerbate BPSD and may expose additional people to harm. Conversely, the current environment may be a significant contributor to BPSD, such that symptoms improve because of a move to a more structured and appropriate environment, and then symptoms return once inpatient treatment is complete. However, an argument can be made for attempting to address as many behavioral problems as possible in the patient's current living situation.

Unfortunately, almost all patients with dementia have a progressive illness. Behavioral and psychological symptoms tend to become more frequent over the course of dementia. Symptoms that have improved or resolved may recur, or new symptoms may appear; some symptoms, such as agitation and apathy, tend to persist over time (van der Linde et al. 2016). Therefore, it is important to set realistic expectations for patients, family members, and other caregivers about the course of BPSD and the likely response to interventions—while offering hope that patients' dignity and quality of life can be preserved for as long as possible and while providing adequate support to caregivers (Brodaty 1999).

A treatment algorithm, incorporating the information in this chapter, is presented in Figure 5–1.

ADDRESSING MEDICAL AND MEDICATION/ SUBSTANCE–RELATED CAUSES

A wide range of medical problems may cause or contribute to BPSD, as discussed in Chapter 4 (see the section "Biological Factors" and Table 4–3). Therefore, the initial step in managing BPSD is to address any identified medical problems. This may involve correcting electrolyte imbalances (e.g., hyponatremia), ensuring adequate hydration and nutrition, and addressing constipation and urinary retention.

Vision and hearing loss are common in patients with dementia and should be corrected. Older adults with hearing loss who do not use hearing aids have higher rates of depression and anxiety than those who do use hearing aids; uncorrected hearing loss has also been associated with cognitive decline (Jorgensen and Messersmith 2015). Patients with dementia who use hearing aids may need help using their hearing aids, can lose their hearing aids, and may be unable to report problems with their hearing aids. On the other hand, the use of hearing aids has been associated with improved speech recognition in patients with dementia and with reduced caregiver distress (Jorgensen and Messersmith 2015). Approximately one-third of patients with AD residing in LTC facilities who have been prescribed eyeglasses do not regularly wear them. Eyeglasses should be labeled to allow for easier identification, patients should have an extra pair of eyeglasses, and patients should get annual or biannual eye exams (Koch et al. 2005).

Unrecognized or untreated pain can precipitate or perpetuate BPSD. As discussed in the section "Identifying and Addressing Pain" in Chapter 2, the prevalence of pain is quite high (47%–68%) in patients with dementia, who in turn may have difficulty reporting or describing their pain (Husebo et al. 2016). A clinician can assess pain in patients with mild or moderate dementia using a 0–10 numerical rating scale or the Iowa Pain Thermometer (viewable online at https://www.painmanagementnursing.org/article/S1524-9042(14)00151-9/pdf) and pain in patients with severe dementia with the Pain Assessment in Advanced Dementia scale (see Table 2–2 in Chapter 2). The most consistently studied and effective intervention for pain is acetaminophen, at dosages up to 3,000 mg/day (Husebo et al. 2016). An alternate approach is a stepwise protocol of treating pain. For example, one effective approach uses acetaminophen up to 3,000 mg/day, extended-release morphine up to 20 mg/day, and/or pregabalin up to 300 mg/day; patients with swallowing difficulties receive a buprenorphine transdermal plaster (Husebo et al. 2014). Tramadol has not been studied in the treat-

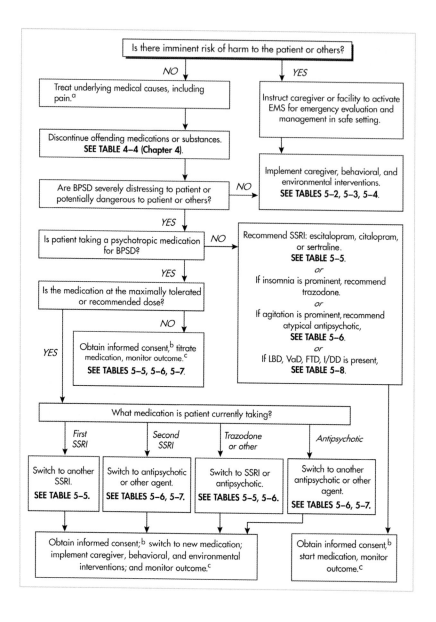

FIGURE 5-1.   Algorithm for responding to behavioral and psychological symptoms of dementia (BPSD) *(opposite page).*

This algorithm presumes that an assessment, as summarized in Figure 4–5 in Chapter 4, has taken place. These are general guidelines and not meant to replace clinical judgment. EMS = emergency medical services; FTD = frontotemporal dementia; I/DD = intellectual/developmental disability; LBD = Lewy body disease (dementia with Lewy bodies or Parkinson disease dementia); SSRI = selective serotonin reuptake inhibitor; VaD = vascular dementia.

[a]Consider adding acetaminophen 1,000 mg two or three times a day, unless contraindicated.

[b]First obtain informed consent from the patient or a proxy decision maker: legal guardian, activated health care power of attorney, or legal next of kin.

[c]Schedule an office visit, telemedicine visit, or phone call in 1 week, with instructions to family or staff to call immediately if BPSD worsen or intolerable side effects occur. Ineffective medications should be discontinued. Even if a medication appears to be effective, consider tapering off slowly after 4–6 months, especially antipsychotics.

ment of pain or behavioral symptoms in patients with dementia, and nonsteroidal anti-inflammatory drugs are best avoided (Husebo et al. 2016). My own recommendation is to consider prescribing acetaminophen 1,000 mg two to three times a day to any patient with BPSD who does not have a history of severe hepatic disease or excess alcohol use; personally, I am wary of recommending an opioid.

As discussed in Chapter 4, there is some controversy about the relationship between urinary tract infections and delirium or BPSD, and there is understandable concern about inappropriate prescription of antibiotics. Antibiotics should certainly not be prescribed empirically for BPSD—rather, the site of infection and pathogen should be identified. Caution should be exercised when selecting an antibiotic: fluoroquinolones, commonly used for pneumonia and urinary tract infections, have been associated with disturbances in attention, disorientation, agitation, anxiety, amnesia, and delirium (U.S. Food and Drug Administration 2018) and therefore are best avoided in older adults with dementia.

Other steps to uncover medical issues include addressing vitamin deficiencies, thyroid dysfunction, obstructive sleep apnea, subdural hematoma, epilepsy, and other conditions listed in Table 4–3.

The clinician should discontinue (or at least reduce dosages of) medications and other substances that could be causing or contributing to BPSD, especially medications with anticholinergic properties, sedative-hypnotic drugs, opioids, and alcohol (see list in Table 4–4). It is especially important to target anticholinergic burden by discontinuing medications that antagonize cholinergic muscarinic receptors. Despite their potential to cause cognitive and psychiatric side effects, anticholinergic medications are commonly prescribed to older adults (Jaïdi et al. 2018). These medications also could antagonize and therefore diminish the benefit from cholinesterase inhibitors used to delay cognitive decline in patients with AD. Medications that contribute significantly to anticholinergic burden include antihistamines, tricyclic antidepressants, paroxetine, antispasmodics (e.g., oxybutynin, dicyclomine), antiparkinsonian agents (specifically, benztropine and trihexyphenidyl), and antipsychotics (including clozapine, olanzapine, and quetiapine). These medications should be either discontinued or replaced with medications without anticholinergic side effects (e.g., replacing paroxetine with escitalopram). Reducing anticholinergic burden reduces the severity and frequency of BPSD and lowers caregiver burden (Jaïdi et al. 2018).

The clinician should keep in mind that it may take several days or even weeks for symptoms to improve after beginning treatment of an underlying medical problem or after discontinuing offending substances.

SUPPORT AND EDUCATION OF FAMILY AND OTHER CAREGIVERS

As depicted in Figure 2–1 in Chapter 2, dementia care involves at least three parties: the patient, the clinician, and the patient's caregiver(s). Supporting and educating patients, family members, and other caregivers is critical to successfully addressing BPSD (Vandepitte et al. 2016). Clinicians should provide family members and other caregivers with a conceptual framework for understanding how BPSD arise and can be managed. The Chapter 3 section "Etiological Models of BPSD" introduced three such frameworks that could prove useful for caregivers:

- The *behavioral model* argues that BPSD arise in response to or following specific antecedents and that the BPSD in turn lead to or are followed by consequences (see Figure 3–2). Behavioral interventions try to decrease the frequency of the unwanted behaviors and increase the frequency of desired, prosocial behaviors.
- The *progressively lowered stress threshold model* posits that BPSD arise from a mismatch between the stressors of the environment and the capacity of a person with dementia to appropriately respond to those stressors (see Figure 3–3). Implementing this model involves the following:
    - Reducing environmental stressors (e.g., reducing noise)
    - Monitoring persons with dementia for early signs of anxiety or agitation

- Compensating for a patient's problems with communication and executive function (e.g., providing a calm and consistent routine)
- Providing unconditional acceptance and positive regard (e.g., using distraction instead of confrontation, using touch to reassure)
- Making allowances for a patient's lowered stress threshold (e.g., by providing rest periods)
- Encouraging caregivers to care for themselves (Smith et al. 2004)
- The *unmet needs model* argues that BPSD may arise because patients are unable to make their needs known and because caregivers have a hard time comprehending those needs (see Figure 3–4). Unmet needs result in a cascade of need-driven, dementia-compromised behaviors, exacerbated by ineffective or counterproductive responses by caregivers (Kovach et al. 2005). On the basis of this framework, caregivers adopt a patient-centered care approach. Specifically, they do the following:
  - Come to understand that BPSD may result from the unmet needs of a person with dementia
  - Communicate with and engage with (rather than avoid or try to control) the person
  - Try to identify the unmet needs that may be resulting in behaviors
  - Address "proximal" (i.e., precipitating) factors such as pain, fatigue, infection, dehydration, and overstimulation (Colling 2004)

Clearly, there is overlap in these approaches. Table 5–2 synthesizes advice to family caregivers, drawn from these various frameworks; the information could easily be turned into a handout for caregivers. Additional resources to educate and support caregivers are listed in the "Resources for Patients, Families, and Caregivers" section later in this chapter.

The caregiver interventions with the greatest efficacy are those that target paid caregivers in LTC settings (Livingston et al. 2014). Interventions for informal caregivers, such as family members, in community settings appear to improve caregivers' confidence in their skills and to decrease caregiver burden (Brasure et al. 2016), but there is mixed evidence about the efficacy of such interventions to reduce patients' BPSD (Brasure et al. 2016; Brodaty and Arasaratnam 2012). Coping strategies such as wishful thinking, denial, and avoidance resulted in worse outcomes for caregivers; interventions should instead emphasize problem-focused coping, acceptance, and social-emotional support (Gilhooly et al. 2016). New approaches that are promising include telehealth (Williams et al. 2018) and structured internet-based interventions (Kales et al. 2018).

TABLE 5–2.   Advice to family caregivers regarding how to respond to behavioral and psychological symptoms of dementia

Category	Advice
General principles	Be flexible and improvise. The behaviors and emotions of the person with dementia can change unexpectedly, so try to "roll with the punches." What worked yesterday may not work today.
	Don't take it personally. Your loved one's behavior and statements are not intentional, manipulative, or meant to be hurtful.
	Allow the person to keep as much control of his or her life as possible. As long as the person is safe, there could be any number of ways of doing things.
	Be realistic about what to expect from your loved one and from yourself. As the disease progresses, he or she will need more help.
Communicating with a person with dementia	Don't try to reason or convince. The person's ability to use logic may not be working properly.
	Try to find the truth or emotion in what the person is saying, and talk about that. For example, if the person fears that food is poisoned, discuss feeling afraid. This is called *validation*.
	Keep your questions, responses, and instructions simple. Don't "overexplain." Avoid open-ended questions. Offer two choices, and you may have to help the person with the choice. Break down instructions into one or two steps at a time.
	Speak more slowly. Allow enough time for the person to respond.
	Use calm, positive statements. Be reassuring and encouraging. Celebrate small successes. Express your gratitude. Try gentle touch.
	Avoid negative words, tone, and facial expressions. Don't ask the person with dementia to "try harder." Don't tell the person that he or she is wrong.
	Take deep breaths and count to 10. Try to stay calm.

TABLE 5–2. Advice to family caregivers regarding how to respond to behavioral and psychological symptoms of dementia *(continued)*

Category	Advice
Maintaining a routine and modifying the environment	Have a routine. Knowing what to expect and when it will happen can be comforting for your loved one. Schedule more challenging activities (e.g., bathing) when the person is likely to be at his or her best.
	Schedule pleasurable activities (e.g., music, singing, dancing). Share a meal with the person's favorite foods. Allow enough time for activities.
	Other activities to consider: walking, talking on the phone, visiting with friends, having a snack, housework, going out to eat, shopping, going to church, praying, or other religious activities.
	Don't overschedule or overstimulate. Reduce clutter, noise, and distractions. If the current location is too distracting, go to another one.
	Schedule meaningful activities. Find ways that the person can contribute (e.g., setting the table, folding laundry). Allow the person to take advantage of his or her remaining social skills.
	Try activities to stimulate the senses: finger paint (using nontoxic paints), pop bubble wrap, build or buy a "busy board," try a "fidget" blanket or other sensory toys.
Caring for the caregiver	Take care of yourself (as advised on airplanes: "Put on your oxygen mask before helping others with their masks").
	Eat healthy foods. Exercise regularly. Don't drink too much alcohol or take mind-altering drugs. Don't drink too much caffeine.
	Make sure to get enough sleep. If your loved one is up at night, you may need to get nighttime help.
	Get routine medical care. When sick, seek medical care.
	Watch for signs of burning out: anxiety, depression, becoming easily angered, trouble sleeping, losing interest or hope, suicidal thinking, poor eating habits, drinking too much alcohol, using mind-altering drugs, trouble concentrating. Get help.

TABLE 5–2. Advice to family caregivers regarding how to respond to behavioral and psychological symptoms of dementia *(continued)*

Category	Advice
Caring for the caregiver *(continued)*	Take regular breaks. Walk away when frustrated or exhausted. Plan respite care regularly.
	Arrange for home care services and adult day care.
	Attend support groups for caregivers. Use online caregiver supports.
	Schedule activities with your friends and family.
Responding to aggression and potentially unsafe behaviors	Watch for early signs of agitation or aggression and respond before things escalate. Keep track of behaviors, and try to identify causes or triggers of the behaviors.
	Don't confront or argue. Don't make sudden movements.
	Try distraction. Shift to another activity. Music may be soothing. The person with dementia might forget what he or she was angry about.
	Give a person who paces a lot of safe space to walk. Make sure he or she is hydrated and eating snacks. Get him or her good shoes.
	Limit access to dangerous items, such as sharp objects and power tools. Remove guns from the home.
	If you or your loved one is unsafe, call emergency services.
Responding to depression and anxiety	Reassure your loved one that he or she is loved and will not be abandoned. Schedule regular activities each day. Have the person spend time with others besides you.
	Reminisce together about pleasant experiences in the past.
	Listen for suicidal statements and get help right away.
Responding to hallucinations and delusions	Don't argue or try to reason. Discuss the underlying emotion, which is usually fear (or maybe anger).

TABLE 5–2. Advice to family caregivers regarding how to respond to behavioral and psychological symptoms of dementia *(continued)*

Category	Advice
Responding to hallucinations and delusions (*continued*)	If the person is stating that an object is missing or has been stolen, try to search for the object. Then talk about another object you found (e.g., a photo album)—that is, use distraction.
	Turn off the television or computer when there are violent or upsetting programs or images.
	If the person is "hearing things" (auditory hallucinations), check for noises that he or she could be misinterpreting.
	If the person is "seeing things" (visual hallucinations), make sure there is adequate lighting. Look for shadows or reflections that the person could be misinterpreting. Cover or remove mirrors (the person could think his or her own reflection is a stranger).
Responding to wandering	Have the person wear a medical identification bracelet. Register him or her with a service such as the Alzheimer's Association MedicAlert + Safe Return program.
	Alert your neighbors and police that your loved one is at risk of wandering. Keep a recent photo on hand.
	Keep house keys and car keys out of sight.
	Consider putting an alarm or bell on the door. Move the lock to be high or low on the door. Add a slide bolt at the top or bottom of the door.
	Schedule activities at the times when your loved one is most likely to wander.
	Make sure your loved one has adequate supervision (e.g., not left alone at home).
	If your loved one elopes, search for no more than 15 minutes and then call emergency services.
Responding to problems with sleep	Schedule enough activities during the day to keep the person busy. Address daytime loneliness and boredom. Encourage your loved one to exercise daily and get enough exposure to light.
	Create a daily routine with the same waking time and bedtime each day.

TABLE 5–2.	Advice to family caregivers regarding how to respond to behavioral and psychological symptoms of dementia *(continued)*

Category	Advice
Responding to problems with sleep *(continued)*	Napping is okay, as long as it is not too late (e.g., 2 P.M. or later) and not too long (more than 1 hour). It may be helpful to schedule one or two rest periods each day.
	If your loved one drinks coffee or tea, switch to decaffeinated versions. The person should avoid drinking alcohol, smoking tobacco, and using mind-altering drugs.
	Before bedtime, create a calm and soothing environment. Turn off the television. Soothing music may help. Read to your loved one.
	Keep a nightlight on in the bedroom, hallways, and bathroom.
	If your loved one is up at night, approach him or her calmly; see if the person needs something; and gently remind him or her that it is bedtime, without arguing.
	You may need help at night (e.g., a paid caregiver or another family member).

Note. These recommendations are intended for family members caring for persons with dementia in their homes; they could also be helpful for family members visiting persons with dementia in long-term care settings.

Source. These recommendations are based on a review and summary of the information provided by the following: Alzheimer's Association (2018), Kales et al. (2014, 2015), National Institute on Aging (2017), and Smith et al. (2004).

Attending support groups can be a critical resource for family caregivers (Vandepitte et al. 2016). Members of caregiver support groups can share knowledge and experiences with each other, such as tips for how to respond to specific behaviors. Participating in a support group can be validating and perhaps reassuring. Support groups may be run by health care professionals or by group members who have received some professional training. Support groups have been found to improve caregivers' mental health (including reducing depression), to reduce caregiver burden, to increase caregivers' social supports, and to improve their relationships with the people for whom they are caring (Chien et al. 2011). In the United States, local chapters of the Alzheimer's Association offer support groups for patients and caregivers.

NONPHARMACOLOGICAL INTERVENTIONS: PSYCHOLOGICAL, BEHAVIORAL, AND ENVIRONMENTAL INTERVENTIONS

All practice guidelines for the treatment of BPSD argue that nonpharmacological interventions should take precedence over pharmacological interventions, primarily due to safety concerns—and that is the position I have adopted. Certainly, the risks of psychotropic medications are higher than the risks of nonpharmacological interventions. Yet, the evidence of efficacy of various nonpharmacological interventions ranges from negative (ineffective relative to control) to insufficient (sample sizes too small or other methodological problems) to modestly positive. Furthermore, nonpharmacological interventions can be difficult to implement—they, after all, do not come in an easy-to-administer pill form. When there is imminent danger to the person with dementia or those around the patient, a nonpharmacological approach may not suffice. Most studies of nonpharmacological interventions have been conducted in LTC settings, and therefore results may not be applicable to patients with dementia who live in their own homes (and, in fact, the majority live in their own homes). Finally, nonpharmacological interventions may inherently be impossible to standardize and may need to be customized for each patient and modified as the patient's illness progresses or circumstances change. Nevertheless, I agree that, except in certain situations, clinicians should recommend nonpharmacological options first.

The most effective nonpharmacological interventions are 1) training and supervising formal (paid) caregivers; 2) implementing structured activities for persons with dementia; 3) music therapy; 4) sensory interventions such as therapeutic touch, massage, and multisensory stimulation; and 5) implementing a dementia care mapping model in nursing homes (see "Long-Term Care Facility" later in this chapter for further discussion of this model) (Legere et al. 2018; Livingston et al. 2014; Scales et al. 2018).

- *Caregiver training:* It is recommended that the staff of facilities caring for persons with dementia be trained in patient-centered care, communication skills, and behavioral principles. Table 5–3 combines elements of these approaches for the purposes of training caregiving staff; staff new to working with persons with dementia may also find the information in Table 5–2 to be helpful. Structured approaches such as DICE, selected by an international Delphi consensus process as the top emerging nonpharmacological treatment for BPSD (Kales et al. 2019), may be most helpful (see the section "Specifying and Characterizing BPSD" in Chapter 4).

- *Structured activities:* Lack of meaningful activities can be a source of frustration and distress for persons with dementia. A wide range of activities have been studied, including storytelling, exercise, gardening, cooking, and Montessori activities (Livingston et al. 2014). Reviews have differed on whether customizing activities for an individual with dementia adds benefit, but such an approach is consistent with patient-centered care (Kales et al. 2019; Scales et al. 2018). Exercise seems to be more helpful for addressing depression than other BPSD (Barreto et al. 2015).

- *Music therapy:* In AD, musical memory is better preserved than verbal memory, so listening to music may evoke pleasant memories and may thereby reduce stress (Scales et al. 2018). To be most effective, music therapy should be led by a trained therapist and should involve a structured program in which patients listen to well-known songs and join in with the music (Livingston et al. 2014). Music therapy is conducted in groups; this prosocial aspect may itself be therapeutic (Scales et al. 2018). Anecdotally, the music that is most enjoyable is the music that the participants listened to in their teens and 20s.

- *Sensory interventions:* Reviews have come to differing conclusions about the effectiveness of *therapeutic touch* (not effective [Livingston et al. 2014]; effective [Legere et al. 2018]; possibly effective, but depends on patient preferences [Scales et al. 2018]). A variety of approaches for massage have been studied, including location (e.g., back, shoulders, neck, hands, lower legs, feet) and method (rubbing or kneading, slow frequency, large amplitude) (Scales et al. 2018). An example of *multisensory stimulation* is Snoezelen, which involves "a dimly lit room that include[s] many objects pertaining to the five senses: fiber-optic cables, aroma therapy, different music/sounds, water columns of different colors, textured balls to touch, and screen projectors" (Brasure et al. 2016, p. C-7). At least some of the benefit from sensory approaches derives from the interaction between patient and therapist (Scales et al. 2018). Sensory interventions have not been rigorously studied in patients' homes, but I suggest that family caregivers consider trying the approaches listed in Table 5–2, under "Maintaining a routine and modifying the environment."

The following psychotherapeutic approaches have some evidence for use in BPSD:

TABLE 5-3. Principles of behavioral management for professional caregivers

Category	Action plan
Practice patient-centered care	The VIPS framework can help staff use a patient-centered care approach: V = *Value* each patient, irrespective of disease and level of functioning. I = *Individual* life story, preferences, and values should inform treatment planning. P = Try to view the situation from the patient's *perspective*. S = *Social* environment (where the patient lives) should be emphasized. Also: • Acknowledge and accept the patient's experience. • Take into consideration the patient's life prior to admission, which may provide clues about current behavior and about effective approaches to care. • Identify past and current hobbies and interests. • Take the patient's report of events, feelings, and thoughts seriously.
Set goals of care	Develop and implement SMART goals: • Specific: State exactly what behavior is being targeted and what the expected outcome is. • Measurable: Determine how the behavior will be assessed and how to determine if the goal has been met. • Achievable: Ensure that the patient and staff can in fact attain the goal. • Relevant: Pick a goal that will have a meaningful impact on the patient. • Time-limited: Determine when the goal should be achieved.

TABLE 5–3.   Principles of behavioral management for professional caregivers *(continued)*

Category	Action plan
Communicate effectively with patients	In addition to the advice to family caregivers in Table 5–2, make sure to do the following: • Give patients enough opportunities and time to express themselves. • Speak in simple and direct language. • Consider using gestures, pictures, written words, or verbal cues.
Promote a regular daily routine	Promote regularity of daily rhythms, including when the patient wakes up, gets medications, eats meals, participates in activities, and goes to bed. • Expose patients to as much daylight (or bright light) as possible during the daytime. If possible, encourage outdoor physical activities. • Encourage physical activities. Promote contacts with other people. Support healthy eating. • Encourage the patient to make his or her own choices in activities and to be as independent as possible with regard to activities of daily living. • Assign staff to work consistently with patients to promote a sense of safety and familiarity. • Schedule activities that the patient will find meaningful, pleasant, and doable. • Ensure that patients, especially those who pace or wander, have adequate hydration and nutrition.
Create a safe and comfortable environment	The environment should feel comfortable and familiar—like a home rather than an institution. • Ensure that each patient has a private space in which he or she can feel safe. Create low-stimulation areas where a patient can rest or take a break. • Ensure sufficient lighting. • Place cues to help patients find their way around the residence. Make sure that areas for dining, activities, and recreation are clearly marked. Make sure that patients have personal furnishings, signs, pictures, or memory boxes to help them recognize their own rooms. • Provide easy, safe, and secure access to the outdoors.

TABLE 5–3. Principles of behavioral management for professional caregivers *(continued)*

Category	Action plan
Create a safe and comfortable environment *(continued)*	• Reduce noise and clutter, such as by eliminating nonemergency overhead paging systems. • Create activity areas with recreational opportunities. • Make exits less obvious to reduce the risk that a patient will wander away from the facility. Use alarms, but not ones that are too obtrusive.

Note. These guidelines are intended for use by professional caregivers (e.g., registered nurses, certified nursing assistants) providing direct care to patients with dementia. Many of the recommendations for family caregivers in Table 5–2 would also be applicable to professional caregivers.
Source. The principles are based on a review and summary of the information provided by the following: Alzheimer's Association (2009), Leontjevas et al. (2013), and Lichtwarck et al. (2017).

- *Reminiscence therapy* appears to be helpful for depression (Gitlin et al. 2012; Scales et al. 2018). This approach "involves discussion of past events and experiences with the aim of increasing well-being and providing pleasure and cognitive stimulation," is predicated on the fact that more remote memories are better preserved than more recent memories (a common finding in dementia due to AD), and can be conducted either individually or in a group (Scales et al. 2018, p. S95).
- *Problem-solving therapy* may be effective for patients with early dementia (or mild cognitive impairment) and depression. This is an individual or group therapy that is used in an attempt to find the best possible solution to current problems (thereby reducing stress) and to teach patients skills to help them solve future problems (Kiosses and Alexopoulos 2014).
- The premise of *validation therapy* is that while the content of what a person with dementia says may not be accurate (e.g., due to amnesia or delusions), the associated emotional experience is real; therefore, rather than focus on content, the caregiver acknowledges and discusses the feelings of the person with dementia (Scales et al. 2018). For example, when a patient reports the paranoid ideation that her purse has been stolen, the caregiver should not challenge the patient on this point but should instead discuss the underlying fear of losing something. Unfortunately, there is insufficient evidence to support the use of validation therapy (Gitlin et al. 2012; Livingston et al. 2014).

- *Simulated presence therapy*, in which video or audio recordings of family members are played for the person with dementia when agitated, has insufficient supporting evidence (Abraha et al. 2017; Livingston et al. 2014).

Most systematic reviews (Brasure et al. 2016; Livingston et al. 2014; Scales et al. 2018), but not all (Gitlin et al. 2012; Legere et al. 2018), have concluded that *aromatherapy* is ineffective for reducing BPSD. *Light therapy* is not effective for reducing agitation or depression (Gitlin et al. 2012; Forbes et al. 2015; Legere et al. 2018; Livingston et al. 2014; Scales et al. 2018). Studies of *pet therapy* (animal-assisted therapy, using either real, stuffed, or robotic animals) have shown promising results but are inconclusive so far (Livingston et al. 2014; Scales et al. 2018).

Nonpharmacological interventions may reduce the use of psychotropic medications. Specifically, implementing a program of cultural change within an LTC facility and focusing on the physicians prescribing medications appear to reduce the prescription of antipsychotic medications (Birkenhäger-Gillesse et al. 2018). Respite care and adult day care programs appear to help reduce behavioral symptoms and may also help improve caregiver outcomes (Vandepitte et al. 2016).

Table 5–4 synthesizes findings regarding psychological, behavioral, and environmental interventions for BPSD.

PHARMACOLOGICAL INTERVENTIONS

In this section, I address when medications should be used to treat BPSD, which medications have the best evidence for efficacy, what safety concerns arise when using medications, and what is the recommended duration of treatment. Jeste et al. (2008) summed up the dilemma of treating BPSD well: "The serious consequences of psychosis and agitation in dementia, the problematic risk-benefit profile of antipsychotic medications for such symptoms, and the paucity of data on other treatment alternatives combine to create a clinical conundrum for which there are no immediate or simple solutions" (p. 966).

Most treatment guidelines recommend that medications, in particular antipsychotic medications, should be used only when BPSD are potentially dangerous to the person with dementia or those around him or her, or when BPSD cause the person with dementia to experience severe distress (e.g., Reus et al. 2016). Whereas the use of antipsychotics has drawn the most attention because of the risk of mortality (and many other side effects), the use of other psychotropic medications, which may be safer but which in general are less effective, is no less complicated.

TABLE 5–4. Principles of psychological, behavioral, and environmental approaches to addressing behavioral and psychological symptoms of dementia

---

The most effective interventions for *patients* are

  Structured activities

  Music therapy

  Sensory interventions

  Reminiscence therapy or problem-solving therapy (for depression)

The most effective intervention for *families* is supporting family caregivers.

The most effective interventions for *facilities* are

  Training programs for formal caregivers

  Dementia care mapping or other quality improvement tools

Each of these interventions will require some investment of resources (e.g., training of staff).

Because no intervention is effective for all patients, an individualized plan should be developed for each person and updated over time as circumstances change.

Specific behaviors should be targeted, and outcomes of interventions should be measured.

Interventions should be culturally sensitive and may need to be tailored to patients' and caregivers' cultural background.

Source. Content based on a review and summary of the information provided by the following: Barrett et al. (2015), Cooper et al. (2010), Legere et al. (2018), Livingston et al. (2014), Scales et al. (2018), and Vandepitte et al. (2016).

After addressing precautions, I review the evidence base for using antidepressants (which are probably safer than antipsychotics but also probably not as effective) and then antipsychotics. I then move on to anticonvulsants (valproate, which is ineffective and poorly tolerated, and carbamazepine, which is possibly effective but may not be well tolerated), benzodiazepines (which are best reserved for emergency, short-term use), cognitive enhancers (which are reasonable for delaying cognitive decline but unlikely to have substantial benefit for BPSD), and other medications (best evidence for pain control, weaker evidence for other medications). Most of the literature pertains to agitation, psychosis, and overall BPSD; I turn later to other BPSD.

Precautions

Prescribing psychotropic medications to persons with dementia requires great caution because of the greater risk of side effects among older adults.

In fact, the Beers list, which inventories medications to be used with caution or not at all in older adults, includes virtually every commonly used psychotropic medication (American Geriatrics Society 2019 Beers Criteria Update Expert Panel 2019). Many protocols have been developed to identify medications of concern, and there is great interest in de-prescribing medications (Barry et al. 2016). In addition to the increased risk of mortality with antipsychotics prescribed to older adults with dementia—which I discuss extensively below—older adults are more likely to experience the following side effects from psychotropic medications:

- Cognitive impairment
- Falls
- Sedation
- Gastrointestinal side effects, including weight loss
- Hyponatremia (with antidepressants)
- Cerebrovascular accidents (with antipsychotics)
- Extrapyramidal symptoms (with antipsychotics)
- Venous thromboembolism (with antipsychotics)

Because polypharmacy is common in older adults, adding a psychotropic medication also raises concern for drug-drug interactions. Clinicians should have a method for identifying potential drug-drug interactions, such as by using a website or smartphone-based app to check interactions.

There are regulatory concerns related to use of psychotropic medications. For example, U.S. federal regulations set restrictions on prescribing psychotropic medications to residents of nursing homes (see the subsection "Long-Term Care Facility" for further discussion), and the U.S. Food and Drug Administration (FDA) has added many warnings to medications—notably, antipsychotics.

Understandably, there has been interest in identifying biomarkers that could help clinicians determine which medication is most likely to be effective and least likely to cause side effects prior to starting treatment. Hope that pharmacogenetic testing can identify such biomarkers is probably premature (Zubenko et al. 2018). There are no studies of using pharmacogenetic testing to determine which medication to use or avoid for BPSD, so there is currently no role for pharmacogenetic testing in caring for persons with dementia.

Antidepressants

Antidepressants may have the best risk-benefit profile of any drug class for pharmacological treatment of BPSD, specifically of agitation and depression. The side-effect burden is lower with antidepressants than with antipsychotics, anticonvulsants, or benzodiazepines. Although the evidence of efficacy is overall somewhat mixed, antidepressants may be most helpful for agitation and less so for depression and anxiety (Farina et al. 2017).

Of the specific antidepressants, citalopram has the strongest evidence for efficacy for agitation, but it is associated with QT prolongation (Farina et al. 2017; Kales et al. 2019). Escitalopram may be effective, without QT prolongation as a side effect and with good cardiac safety. Both citalopram and escitalopram are unlikely to have significant drug-drug interactions. After initial promise for sertraline for treating depression, more recent trials have not demonstrated efficacy (Farina et al. 2017); this is unfortunate, because sertraline has minimal drug-drug interactions and good cardiac safety. Fluoxetine has not been found to be effective for BPSD, has a long half-life, and has the potential for drug-drug interactions. Paroxetine and tricyclic antidepressants should be avoided because of their anticholinergic properties. Venlafaxine has not been found to be effective for BPSD, can raise blood pressure, and can be difficult to wean off due to serotonin withdrawal. Duloxetine has not been studied except in DLB.

Outside of the context of dementia, venlafaxine and duloxetine have been found to be modestly helpful for neuropathic pain. Mirtazapine occupies an important niche in the treatment of older adults with depression because of its positive effects on sleep and appetite, but trials in BPSD have thus far been negative (Farina et al. 2017). Vortioxetine may improve cognition in older adults with major depressive disorder, but it has not yet been tested in dementia.

Bupropion has not been studied well in dementia, and it should be used with caution given the associated risk of seizures. It is the antidepressant least likely to cause hyponatremia (see following discussion of this side effect). Bupropion has typically been used to treat depression when anergia or amotivation is a prominent symptom; on the other hand, it should be used with caution in patients with insomnia, weight loss, anxiety, or seizures because these are potential side effects.

Trazodone has a good evidence base in the treatment of BPSD due to FTD; though not formally studied in BPSD due to other causes, trazodone may certainly be a reasonable option, especially for insomnia.

Discontinuing antidepressants in patients with AD and vascular dementia is associated with worsening depressive symptoms and overall BPSD, underscoring that they in fact have therapeutic value (Bergh et al. 2012).

Almost all antidepressants can cause hyponatremia, presumably through a SIADH (syndrome of inappropriate antidiuretic hormone secretion)–like mechanism (De Picker et al. 2014; Viramontes et al. 2016). Bupropion is an exception; mirtazapine may have a risk that is lower than the selective serotonin reuptake inhibitors (SSRIs) and serotonin-norepinephrine reuptake inhibitors (SNRIs) but higher than bupropion; interestingly, trazodone may also have lower risk of hyponatremia despite being serotonergic. Risk factors for antidepressant-induced hyponatremia include age 65 years or older, female sex, and coprescription with diuretics. Hyponatremia usually arises 2–3 weeks after starting an antidepressant or 2–3 weeks after titration. My own experience is that a patient's plasma sodium level will decrease by 2–3 mg/dL after starting or titrating an antidepressant (other than bupropion); whether this is clinically significant depends on the patient's baseline sodium level and medical comorbidities. If hyponatremia develops with one SSRI or SNRI, it is likely to occur with other SSRIs or SNRIs. (Note that most of this information comes from the literature on treating depressed or anxious older adults without dementia.)

My practice is to check a patient's baseline plasma sodium level and to check again 2–3 weeks after starting a medication and 2–3 weeks after each dosage increase. If the baseline sodium level is below normal, I may consider using bupropion, mirtazapine, trazodone, or another drug class. If the patient has a good response to an antidepressant but hyponatremia has developed, I may recommend that the patient add a salt tablet to his or her diet or have at least one drink per day that is high in sodium (e.g., a vegetable juice), unless there is a contraindication to a high-sodium diet.

All psychotropic medications, including antidepressants, can increase the risk of falls. Therefore, patients at risk of falling should be monitored closely for gait imbalance when starting an antidepressant.

The most common side effects of antidepressants are gastrointestinal: stomach upset, nausea, constipation, diarrhea, anorexia, and weight loss (except that mirtazapine can cause weight gain). Persons with dementia may not be able to report these side effects, which may, instead, manifest as (worsening) agitation. Weight loss is of particular concern in older adults because they may already be underweight; losing muscle mass can contribute to debilitation and disability. Antidepressants can cause a wide range of other side effects relevant to patients with BPSD, including sedation, insomnia, changes in rapid eye movement (REM) sleep, restlessness, anxiety, and impaired cognition—in fact, one study found that 94% of subjects receiving antidepressants developed a side effect (Farina et al. 2017).

Interestingly, a large retrospective study of mortality associated with psychotropic medications found a small but statistically significant increase in mortality over the first 180 days of treatment in patients who received antidepressants compared with those who did not (8.3% vs. 8.0%), yielding a number needed to harm (NNH) of 166 (Maust et al. 2015). This finding has not yet been replicated or clearly explained, though perhaps QT prolongation associated with citalopram may be partially responsible. (See the next subsection, "Antipsychotics," for further discussion of NNH in general and of the Maust et al. [2015] study in particular.)

Table 5–5 includes additional details regarding the use of antidepressants (specifically, SSRIs and trazodone) for BPSD, and Figure 5–1 shows the place of antidepressants in a treatment algorithm. My recommendation is to start with escitalopram; if ineffective or not tolerated, citalopram or sertraline could be considered. If SSRIs are not effective or tolerated, or if insomnia is the most prominent BPSD, I consider a trial of trazodone—see dosing information in the "Frontotemporal Dementia" subsection (later in chapter). Other antidepressants have limited roles for depression and no role in agitation: mirtazapine could be considered if insomnia or weight loss is prominent; bupropion if hyponatremia has prevented the use of other antidepressants or if apathy is prominent; and duloxetine or venlafaxine if neuropathic pain is suspected (based on evidence for patients without dementia). Tricyclic antidepressants should be avoided because of anticholinergic side effects (including worsening cognition) and overall poor tolerability in older adults with dementia.

Antipsychotics

The most controversial topic in the care of patients with BPSD is the use of antipsychotic medications. Antipsychotics have the largest evidence base (in terms of number of studies and subjects of those studies) of any intervention for BPSD, pharmacological or nonpharmacological. Randomized controlled trials (RCTs) indicate that antipsychotics have modest efficacy in reducing agitation and psychosis (pooled effect size of 0.18) (Jeste et al. 2008), though I believe that the sense of most clinicians and formal caregivers is that antipsychotics are quite effective. On the other hand, antipsychotics are associated with increased mortality, resulting in an FDA black box warning advising against the use of antipsychotics in older adults with dementia. This section provides the data on efficacy and side effects of antipsychotics in BPSD and recommendations regarding their use.

Efficacy

The antipsychotics with the clearest evidence of efficacy for BPSD are the atypical antipsychotics (also known as second-generation antipsychotics) risperidone, olanzapine, and aripiprazole. An Agency for Healthcare Research and Quality Comparative Effectiveness Review found that risperidone is effective for psychosis, agitation, and overall BPSD; olanzapine is most effective for agitation, less so for overall BPSD, and equivocal for psychosis; aripiprazole is effective for overall BPSD and less so for psychosis and

TABLE 5–5. Using antidepressants to address behavioral and psychological symptoms of dementia

Medication	Dosing	Comments
Bupropion	Start once-daily extended-release (XL) formulation 150 mg at breakfast, then increase to 300 mg at breakfast; after 4 weeks, consider increasing to maximum dosage of 450 mg at breakfast.	Very limited data on use in dementia; side effects can include seizures, insomnia, weight loss, anxiety, agitation; avoid in patients with epilepsy, head injury, electrolyte disturbances; the antidepressant least likely to cause hyponatremia.
Citalopram (*first-line agent*)	Start 10 mg at breakfast for 1 week, then increase to 20 mg at breakfast; after 4 weeks, may increase to 30 mg at breakfast, but will require electrocardiogram; may require 9 weeks for full response.	**FDA black box warning regarding risk of QT prolongation associated with dosage > 20 mg/day in those older than age 60 years.**
Duloxetine	Start 20 mg at breakfast for 1 week, then increase to 40 mg at breakfast; after 4 weeks, may increase to maximum dosage of 60 mg at breakfast.	Only one unpublished trial of duloxetine for depression in Lewy body disease; avoid in patients with liver disease or excess alcohol consumption.
Escitalopram (*first-line agent*)	Start 5 mg at breakfast for 1 week, then increase to 10 mg at breakfast; after 4 weeks, may increase to 15 mg at breakfast; after another 4 weeks, may increase to maximum dosage of 20 mg at breakfast.	Unclear if FDA black box warning regarding citalopram also applies to escitalopram; may be prudent to monitor QT interval at dosages above 10 mg/day.
Fluoxetine	Start 10 mg at breakfast for 1 week, then increase to 20 mg at breakfast; may increase to maximum dosage of 40 mg at breakfast after 4 weeks.	Potential for drug-drug interactions; studies in dementia have been negative.

TABLE 5–5. Using antidepressants to address behavioral and psychological symptoms of dementia *(continued)*

Medication	Dosing	Comments
Mirtazapine	Start 15 mg at bedtime and continue for 4 weeks; may increase to 30 mg at bedtime for 4 weeks, then maximum dosage of 45 mg at bedtime; consider starting at 7.5 mg at bedtime if concern about tolerability.	Common side effects include sedation and increased appetite, which may be helpful for insomnia; clinical trials for depression in dementia have been negative.
Paroxetine	*Recommend against use in dementia because of anticholinergic side effects and risk of worsening cognition.*	
Sertraline *(first-line agent in patients with cardiac disease)*	Start 25 mg at breakfast for 1 week, then increase to 50 mg at breakfast; after 4 weeks, may increase to 100 mg at breakfast; after another 4 weeks, may increase to maximum dosage of 150 mg at breakfast.	After initially positive studies, more recent studies have been negative; safer than citalopram in patients with cardiac disease.
Trazodone	Start 25–50 mg at bedtime; may titrate by 50-mg/day increments as tolerated, up to a maximum of 250 mg/day; usually dosed at night, but could consider dividing into two to three doses per day.	Monitor for orthostatic hypotension, excess sedation, falls; strongest evidence for efficacy is in FTD, though there is some evidence of effectiveness for insomnia in AD.
Tricyclic antidepressants	*Recommend against use in dementia because of anticholinergic side effects, risk of worsening cognition, and QT prolongation.*	

TABLE 5–5. Using antidepressants to address behavioral and psychological symptoms of dementia *(continued)*

Medication	Dosing	Comments
Venlafaxine	Start once-daily extended-release (XR) formulation 37.5 mg at breakfast for 1 week, then increase to 75 mg at breakfast; after 4 weeks, may increase to 150 mg at breakfast; after another 4 weeks, may increase to maximum dosage of 225 mg at breakfast.	Monitor blood pressure; gastrointestinal side effects may be especially common; discontinuation can be difficult due to serotonin withdrawal symptoms; little evidence supporting efficacy in dementia.

Note.   Medications are listed in alphabetical order; only antidepressants that have been studied in subjects with dementia are included. All antidepressants except bupropion carry risk of hyponatremia in older adults, especially women and those taking diuretics.
AD=Alzheimer's disease; FDA=U.S. Food and Drug Administration; FTD=frontotemporal dementia.

agitation (Maglione et al. 2011). Despite widespread clinical use, quetiapine has consistently failed to outperform placebo with respect to reducing agitation, psychosis, and overall BPSD (Reus et al. 2016); it may have a role in Lewy body disease, though even in that use the evidence for efficacy is weak. Clozapine has an important role in the treatment of psychosis associated with Lewy body disease, but few data have been reported regarding its use for other BPSD and other causes of dementia. Both quetiapine and clozapine are discussed later in this chapter in regard to the treatment of patients with Lewy body disease. Haloperidol, the best studied typical (or first-generation) antipsychotic, appears to be as effective as atypical antipsychotics for BPSD, but it has even more severe safety concerns (Reus et al. 2016). Few head-to-head trials have been reported among the aforementioned atypical antipsychotics (those studies that exist indicate no difference in efficacy), and there are no published trials of other atypical antipsychotics (i.e., asenapine, brexpiprazole, cariprazine, iloperidone, lurasidone, paliperidone, ziprasidone) for BPSD (Reus et al. 2016).

Treatment response typically comes within 2–4 weeks (Schneider et al. 2006a). As noted, even the antipsychotics most likely to be effective have unimpressive effect sizes. The number needed to treat ranges from 5 to 14 (Jeste et al. 2008); in other words, out of every 5–14 patients whose BPSD improve, improvement is due to the effect of the medication in only 1 patient, whereas other factors account for improvement in the other 4–13 patients.

Why do medications that in clinical practice seem to be so effective fare so poorly in RCTs? The placebo response rate is high in many trials of antipsychotics for agitation and psychosis. BPSD wax and wane, so improvement may simply be due to the passage of time. Some improvement may be due to regression to the mean. Finally, subjects in the placebo arm of clinical trials may get increased attention and other nonspecific treatment effects from interactions with study personnel (Schneider et al. 2006a). In clinical practice, the benefit that many, if not most, patients apparently get from antipsychotics may be due to something other than the psychotropic effects of these medications, including the tincture of time. These observations also apply to placebo response in antidepressant trials (Rosenberg et al. 2015).

Side Effects

Antipsychotics are associated with increased mortality, a finding which led the FDA in 2005 to issue this black box warning: "Elderly patients with dementia-related psychosis treated with antipsychotic drugs are at an increased risk of death." Schneider et al. (2005) published the seminal study that discovered this link. They analyzed 15 trials consisting of 5,110 subjects with dementia randomized to receive either antipsychotic or placebo over the course of 10–12 weeks. Their primary finding was that the odds ratio of mortality in subjects exposed to antipsychotic versus placebo was 1.54, with a 95% confidence interval of 1.06 to 2.23—in other words, a roughly 50% relative increase in mortality. In terms of raw numbers, 3.5% of subjects receiving antipsychotics died, whereas 2.3% of subjects receiving placebo died. The risk difference was 0.01, resulting in an NNH of 100: for every 100 patients with dementia treated with antipsychotic, there will be one additional death associated with antipsychotic use.

Multiple studies since 2005 have confirmed and refined this finding. For example, a retrospective study of 90,786 U.S. veterans age 65 years or older with a diagnosis of dementia found a higher risk of death during the first 180 days of treatment, relative to placebo, with haloperidol and risperidone (NNH of 26 and 27, respectively) than with olanzapine and quetiapine (NNH of 40 and 50, respectively) (Maust et al. 2015). There appeared to be a relationship between the dosage of antipsychotic used and the risk of mortality. Note that the higher risk reported in this study compared with Schneider et al. (2005) may be due to its observational, retrospective nature, which introduces the possibility of confounding by indication (i.e., sicker patients may have been more likely to receive an antipsychotic; therefore, underlying illness may have increased their risk of dying). I view the Maust et al. (2015) findings as confirmatory and, with patients and families, I cite the Schneider et al. (2005) numbers as probably more directly relevant. Given that the risk appears to be highest for haloperidol, I recommend avoiding this medication except in emergency situations.

What accounts for this increase in mortality? The two most plausible explanations are cardiac complications of QT interval prolongation and pneumonia. Most antipsychotics, including ziprasidone, risperidone, haloperidol, olanzapine, and quetiapine, can cause QT prolongation; aripiprazole is not associated with QT prolongation (Leucht et al. 2013). QT prolongation in turn is a risk factor for torsades de pointes and therefore cardiac mortality. Older adults prescribed antipsychotics had a 60% increase in risk of developing pneumonia relative to those not prescribed antipsychotics, with the highest risk during the first week (Knol et al. 2008); presumably, sedation from antipsychotics increases the risk of aspiration pneumonia, which in turn increases risk of dying. As detailed later in this subsection, antipsychotics are also associated with a host of other side effects that could increase mortality, including stroke, venous thromboembolism, and falls.

The higher risk of dying does not seem to abate after 3–6 months and may persist for up to 3 years. In a study randomizing persons with dementia to either continue taking the antipsychotic they had been prescribed or discontinue it, the probability of surviving the first year was 70% in the former group and 77% in the latter group; at 2 years, survival was 46% versus 71%, and at 3 years, 30% versus 59% (Ballard et al. 2009). Discontinuing antipsychotic use after only 3 months of treatment has typically *not* been associated with worsening BPSD, except in patients with more severe baseline BPSD (Van Leeuwen et al. 2018).

Many other side effects can arise. During the seminal Clinical Antipsychotic Trials of Intervention Effectiveness–Alzheimer's Disease (CATIE-AD) study comparing risperidone, olanzapine, and quetiapine to placebo in AD, 63% of subjects had discontinued the medication they had been initially prescribed due to side effects by week 12 (Schneider et al. 2006b). The following are side effects other than mortality:

- *Sedation:* Sedation is among the most common side effects of antipsychotics (and psychotropic medications) in elderly patients. Risperidone, quetiapine, olanzapine, and even aripiprazole are all more likely to cause sedation than placebo (20% for all antipsychotics vs. 8% for placebo) (Reus et al. 2016). In fact, the therapeutic effect of antipsychotics may be due in part to sedation. Taking the antipsychotic at night, avoiding daytime doses, and keeping the total daily dosage low may decrease sedation.
- *Cognitive decline:* Antipsychotics can exacerbate underlying cognitive impairment, either through sedation, anticholinergic effects (e.g., quetiapine has a metabolite, norquetiapine, that is anticholinergic; olanzapine may have anticholinergic properties as well), or other mechanisms. In the CATIE-AD study, antipsychotics were associated with the equivalent of 1 year's worth of cognitive deterioration, and therefore, they potentially offset any benefit from cognitive enhancers (Vigen et al. 2011).
- *Extrapyramidal symptoms (EPS):* Parkinsonism is prevalent among older adults at baseline, and many patients with BPSD have either Parkinson disease dementia (PDD) or DLB. Most antipsychotics can cause or exacerbate tremor, bradykinesia, and rigidity (Reus et al. 2016). Although the literature is not entirely consistent, I would rank the antipsychotics as follows with respect to the propensity to cause or exacerbate EPS: haloperidol > risperidone > aripiprazole > olanzapine > quetiapine = clozapine. The risk of EPS with quetiapine and clozapine is no higher than with placebo. Also, if agitation worsens after a patient starts taking an antipsychotic, the clinician should consider the possibility that akathisia is the cause. Older adults with psychotic disorders are much more likely to develop tardive dyskinesia when taking antipsychotics than are younger

adults, with typical antipsychotics conferring higher risk than atypical antipsychotics (Jeste et al. 1999). This risk of tardive dyskinesia has not been well studied in persons with dementia.

- *Falls, fractures:* Falls are a significant worry for older adults. Dementia itself, BPSD, and psychotropic medications all increase the risk of falls. In their review of the literature, the authors of "The American Psychiatric Association Practice Guideline on the Use of Antipsychotics to Treat Agitation or Psychosis in Patients With Dementia" (Reus et al. 2016) conclude that antipsychotics increase the risk of falls and fractures by 1.5–2.5 times. For nursing home residents, wandering is a risk factor for falling, and it is possible that an antipsychotic could *reduce* the risk of falling by decreasing wandering (Katz et al. 2004), though I am cautious about applying this finding too enthusiastically. When a new psychotropic medication is started, however, the patient should be monitored for increased gait instability.

- *Metabolic complications, including weight gain:* Olanzapine is the most likely antipsychotic to cause weight gain in persons with dementia, with less strong evidence for this side effect with risperidone and quetiapine (Reus et al. 2016); note that in some circumstances, weight gain could be a desirable outcome. The risk of hyperglycemia and dyslipidemia in persons with dementia is unclear (Reus et al. 2016).

- *Stroke:* The Agency for Healthcare Research and Quality Comparative Effectiveness Review found that risperidone was associated with an increased risk of stroke relative to placebo (2.2% vs. 1.1%), yielding an NNH of 53 (Reus et al. 2016). A subsequent study also found an increased risk with use of olanzapine (Reus et al. 2016). Some, but not all, antipsychotics have received FDA labeling regarding a heightened risk of stroke. The risk of stroke appears to be highest in the first month of use. Reus et al. (2016) argue that the overall evidence of risk of stroke is low, and it is unclear if vascular disease increases the risk.

- *Venous thromboembolism:* Atypical antipsychotics may increase the risk of venous thromboembolism, but the evidence has not been consistent, and it is therefore difficult to determine risk with any precision (Jönsson et al. 2018).

- *Prolactin:* In persons with dementia, risperidone has been associated with increased prolactin levels (Reus et al. 2016), which in turn can cause gynecomastia or galactorrhea or have a deleterious effect on bone density. In patients with schizophrenia, aripiprazole has been added to risperidone to lower elevated prolactin levels, but I recommend against this sort of polypharmacy in older adults.

- *Cardiovascular events:* There may be a higher risk of cardiovascular events, including edema, with use of risperidone and olanzapine (Reus et al. 2016).
- *Neutropenia:* Although neutropenia has been found to be a side effect of many antipsychotics, this is chiefly a concern with the use of clozapine, which can cause agranulocytosis. See the subsection "Lewy Body Disease" later in this chapter for further discussion of clozapine's side effects.

For older adults, I recommend avoiding intramuscular injections of antipsychotics, especially long-acting depot formulations (except in patients with chronic psychotic disorders) (Reus et al. 2016). Finally, it is unclear what the risks associated with antipsychotic use are in patients with chronic psychotic disorders who go on to develop dementia (Reus et al. 2016).

Recommendations

See Table 5–6 for additional details regarding the use of antipsychotics for BPSD and Figure 5–1, earlier in chapter, for the place of antipsychotics in a treatment algorithm. I recommend starting with risperidone (or aripiprazole if QT prolongation is a concern), unless the patient has parkinsonism or Lewy body disease. If the patient has parkinsonism (but does not have PDD or DLB), I start with olanzapine. If the patient has PDD or DLB, quetiapine is usually the first-line agent (despite the weak evidence for efficacy), followed by clozapine (see the later subsection "Lewy Body Disease" for further discussion). I find that there is very little role for any other antipsychotic, especially typical antipsychotics. Titration should be slow, and the lowest effective dosage should be found.

Informed consent entails a discussion with the proxy decision maker (e.g., legal next of kin, activated health care power of attorney, legal guardian) regarding the benefits and the risks of atypical antipsychotics, including the risk of mortality. I present decision makers with the data from the Schneider et al. (2005) study—namely, that the risk of dying within the first 10–12 weeks was 3.5% for antipsychotics versus 2.3% for placebo. I discuss the need for careful monitoring for sedation, falls, parkinsonism, and other side effects; for metabolic monitoring; and, if indicated, for monitoring the QT interval via serial electrocardiograms. The authors of the American Psychiatric Association practice guideline (Reus et al. 2016) noted, "Monitoring blood pressure, weight, body mass index (BMI), waist circumference, fasting glucose, fasting lipid profile, and personal/family history have been suggested at baseline for individuals receiving antipsychotic medication, with additional personal/family history and waist circumference annually, blood pressure and fasting plasma glucose at 12 weeks

TABLE 5–6.   Using antipsychotics to address behavioral and psychological symptoms of dementia

Medication	Dosing	Cautions (in addition to risk of mortality)
Aripiprazole (*first-line agent*)	Start 2.5 mg at bedtime, increase to 5 mg at bedtime after 1 week; may increase to 7.5 mg at bedtime after 2–4 weeks, and again to maximum dosage of 10 mg at bedtime after another 2–4 weeks.	More likely to cause EPS than clozapine, olanzapine, and quetiapine; perhaps less sedating than other antipsychotics; unlikely to cause QT prolongation; long half-life could be a problem if patient has intolerable side effects, but could be an advantage if patient intermittently refuses or forgets to take medication.
Clozapine	Start 6.25–12.5 mg at bedtime; titrate slowly to dosage of 25–50 mg at bedtime or divide into twice-daily dosing.	Requires monitoring of absolute neutrophil count; side effects include sedation, sialorrhea, dry mouth, constipation; caution in patients with cardiac disease. See text for full warnings regarding clozapine.
Haloperidol	Start 0.5 mg once daily and titrate with caution; recommend against use except in emergency situations with appropriate medical monitoring.	Highest risk of mortality among antipsychotics; highest risk of EPS; highest risk of QT prolongation.
Olanzapine (*first-line agent*)	Start 2.5 mg at bedtime, increase to 5 mg at bedtime after 1 week; may increase to 7.5 mg at bedtime after 2–4 weeks, and again to maximum dosage of 10 mg at bedtime after another 2–4 weeks; may be divided into twice-daily dosing.	Moderate risk of EPS; quite sedating and appetite stimulating.

TABLE 5–6. Using antipsychotics to address behavioral and psychological symptoms of dementia *(continued)*

Medication	Dosing	Cautions (in addition to risk of mortality)
Quetiapine *(first-line agent in patients with parkinsonism)*	Start 25 mg at bedtime and increase by 25 mg/day every 2–4 weeks; may be divided into twice-daily dosing; target dosage of 100–200 mg/day.	Effective dosages may not be tolerated due to sedation, falls, cognitive impairment; least likely to cause EPS (other than clozapine), and so may be first choice in Lewy body disease.
Risperidone *(first-line agent)*	Start 0.25 mg at bedtime, increase to 0.5 mg at bedtime after 1 week, may increase to 1 mg at bedtime or 0.5 mg twice daily.	Dosages greater than 1 mg/day associated with EPS; avoid in patients with Lewy body disease.

Note. Only antipsychotics that have been studied in subjects with dementia are included. They are listed in alphabetical order.
In the United States, all antipsychotics have a black box label indicating that they should not be used in elderly patients with dementia, due to the risk of mortality. Antipsychotics should be prescribed only after very careful review of risks, benefits, and alternatives.
EPS = extrapyramidal symptoms.

and annually, lipid profile at 12 weeks and every 5 years, and weight with calculation of BMI monthly for 3 months, then quarterly" (pp. 18–19). My own practice is similar to this guidance, though I am not sure there is much value in glucose and lipid monitoring in persons with advanced dementia.

The practice guideline recommends that "if there is no clinically significant response after a 4-week trial of an adequate dose of an antipsychotic drug, the medication should be tapered and withdrawn" (Reus et al. 2016, p. 4). In such a case, I recommend reassessing the situation and determining again whether a medication is indicated and, if so, whether this should be another antipsychotic, an antidepressant, or another agent. I give the same advice for patients experiencing significant side effects.

The long-term goal should be discontinuation of an antipsychotic. For patients who have had a clinically significant response to an antipsychotic, the practice guideline recommends that "an attempt to taper and withdraw the drug should be made within 4 months of initiation, unless the patient experienced a recurrence of symptoms with prior attempts at tapering of antipsychotic medication" (Reus et al. 2016, p. 4). This recommendation is consistent with U.S. regulations requiring a gradual dosage reduction after 6 months, or documentation as to why reduction is not indicated. In principle, I agree, though in practice I have found it difficult to convince family members or caregivers at residential facilities that this an appropriate course of action, particularly when they perceive the medication as having been very helpful. If a decision is made to taper the medication, the taper should take place slowly and with enough time between reductions to determine outcome; the duration of the taper should be proportional to the severity of initial symptoms. For example, when tapering off risperidone 1 mg/day, I suggest decreasing by 0.25–0.5 mg/day every 2–4 weeks. The practice guideline very reasonably recommends that "assessment of symptoms should occur at least monthly during the taper and for at least 4 months after medication discontinuation to identify signs of recurrence" (Reus et al. 2016, p. 4).

Anticonvulsants

The anticonvulsant with the strongest evidence of efficacy for BPSD is carbamazepine (Konovalov et al. 2008); in one treatment algorithm, carbamazepine is recommended ahead of citalopram (Davies et al. 2018). I believe, however, that the significant potential for drug-drug interactions (carbamazepine is a potent inducer of cytochrome P450 enzymes) and the long list of side effects (including neutropenia, hyponatremia, liver failure, and Stevens-Johnson syndrome) limit its usefulness—therefore, I would place carbamazepine behind citalopram in a treatment algorithm for BPSD.

Valproate is not effective for BPSD, has significant side effects, and has been associated with accelerated hippocampal and global atrophy (Fleisher et al. 2011; Lonergan and Luxenberg 2009). I do not recommend its use. Oxcarbazepine does not appear to be effective for BPSD. One small trial, not placebo controlled, of topiramate found it as effective as risperidone for agitation and overall BPSD; I would not recommend using topiramate given its potential for worsening cognition. A small open-label trial of lamotrigine found modest evidence of benefit for agitation. There are only case reports and case series describing benefit from gabapentin but no clinical trials; it would be reasonable to consider a trial of gabapentin, as described in Table 5–7, if other agents (antidepressants, antipsychotics) have failed or not been tolerated.

Although epilepsy is not uncommon among persons with dementia, the literature regarding the use of anticonvulsants is very limited. Levetiracetam may worsen mood in patients with AD and epilepsy; lamotrigine could improve mood but worsen cognition (Liu et al. 2016). See Table 5–7 for a summary regarding the use of anticonvulsants.

Benzodiazepines

Despite the widespread use of benzodiazepines in older adults, the evidence demonstrating efficacy for BPSD is very limited (Tampi and Tampi 2014). Benzodiazepines have been associated with falls, fractures, cognitive impairment, and tolerance in older adults. The authors of a treatment algorithm for BPSD recommend slowly tapering off benzodiazepines and "z-drugs" (eszopiclone, zaleplon, zolpidem) "unless there is clear recent evidence of insurmountable difficulty in stopping them" (Davies et al. 2018, p. 514). The same authors concluded that "occasional use of the benzodiazepine lorazepam as a PRN [as needed] drug was acceptable in cases of extreme agitation or aggression where behavioral interventions and trazodone are ineffective or when brief stressful circumstances might exacerbate or induce agitation and aggression, for example, medical tests or dental procedures" (Davies et al. 2018, p. 514). Among the benzodiazepines, lorazepam is likely the safest because it is metabolized only via glucuronidation; most other benzodiazepines are also metabolized via oxidative metabolism, which is more prone to the effects of aging. Clonazepam for REM sleep behavior disorder is reasonable (see subsection "Disturbances of Sleep").

Cognitive Enhancers

Cholinesterase inhibitors have little if any benefit for BPSD (Wang et al. 2015), except in patients with Lewy body disease. They may also contribute

TABLE 5–7. Other pharmacological approaches to behavioral and psychological symptoms of dementia (BPSD)

Medication	Dosing	Cautions
Acetaminophen (*consider for all patients who may have pain*)	1,000 mg two or three times a day.	Avoid in patients with hepatic disease or significant alcohol consumption.
Carbamazepine	Start 100 mg at bedtime; increase by 100 mg/day weekly; target blood level of 5–8 μg/mL.	Monitor drug level, absolute neutrophil count, sodium, liver function tests; high potential for drug-drug interactions.
Clonazepam	Start 0.5 mg at bedtime; if not effective, may increase to 1 mg at bedtime.	Use only for patients with REM sleep behavior disorder; monitor for sedation, falls, cognitive impairment, disinhibition, respiratory suppression.
Dextromethorphan-quinidine (*second-line agent*)	Start 20/10 mg of dextromethorphan-quinidine in the morning; after 1 week, increase to two times a day; after another 2 weeks, increase to 30/10 mg two times a day.	Most common side effects were falls, diarrhea, UTI, and dizziness; monitor for cardiac side effects; mean increase of QT interval was 5 milliseconds (Cummings et al. 2015).
Donepezil and other cholinesterase inhibitors	For donepezil, start 5 mg at breakfast; after 1 month, increase to 10 mg at breakfast; dosage of 23 mg/day is unlikely to offer additional benefit; consider starting at 2.5 mg at breakfast if tolerability is a concern.	Can cause or exacerbate insomnia, weight loss, hallucinations, bradycardia, falls; do not dose in the evening because may cause insomnia or nightmares.

TABLE 5–7. Other pharmacological approaches to behavioral and psychological symptoms of dementia (BPSD) *(continued)*

Medication	Dosing	Cautions
Gabapentin	Dosages of 200–1,200 mg/day have been reported in case series; consider starting at 100 mg at bedtime or 100 mg two times a day and titrating by 100 mg/day weekly.	Monitor for dizziness, sedation, and gait instability; very limited evidence to support efficacy.
Lorazepam	Recommend against use except in emergency situations or to reduce anxiety for procedures.	Monitor for sedation, falls, cognitive impairment, disinhibition, respiratory suppression.
Melatonin	1–3 mg 2–3 hours before bedtime.	Low potential for side effects but also unlikely to be effective for insomnia in dementia; may be helpful for REM sleep behavior disorder.
Memantine	Once-daily formulation: 7 mg/day for 1 week, then 14 mg/day for 1 week, then 21 mg/day for 1 week, then 28 mg/day thereafter. Twice-daily formulation: 5 mg in morning for 1 week, then 5 mg two times a day for 1 week, then 10 mg in the morning and 5 mg at bedtime for 1 week, then 10 mg two times a day thereafter.	Generally well tolerated; unlikely to have much benefit for BPSD but perhaps less likely than cholinesterase inhibitors to cause or exacerbate BPSD.

TABLE 5–7. Other pharmacological approaches to behavioral and psychological symptoms of dementia (BPSD) (*continued*)

Medication	Dosing	Cautions
Methylphenidate (*use only in patients with apathy*)	Start 5 mg two times a day (morning and noon); after 2 weeks, may titrate to 10 mg two times a day (morning and noon).	Monitor blood pressure and heart rate; avoid in patients with cardiac arrhythmias; can cause weight loss and insomnia.
Pimavanserin (*use only in patients with psychosis due to Parkinson disease*)	34 mg/day is both the initial and the target dosage.	May be associated with higher risk of mortality; can cause QT prolongation; potential for drug-drug interactions; mixed data on efficacy.
Prazosin (*second-line agent*)	Start 1 mg at bedtime, titrating by 1 mg/day weekly up to a maximum of 2 mg in the morning and 4 mg at bedtime.	Monitor for dizziness, falls, sedation, and hypotension.
Valproate	Not recommended due to risk of side effects, including brain atrophy.	

Note.   Only medications other than antidepressants and antipsychotics that have been studied in subjects with dementia are included. They are listed in alphabetical order.

REM=rapid eye movement; UTI=urinary tract infection.

to BPSD by causing or exacerbating insomnia, hallucinations, gastrointestinal distress, muscle cramps, or depression. Memantine is ineffective for BPSD (Ballard et al. 2015; Wang et al. 2015). Therefore, I would not recommend cognitive enhancers to specifically address BPSD, except in Lewy body disease (discussed later).

As reviewed in Chapter 2 (see the subsection "Pharmacological Approaches" and Table 2–1), cognitive enhancers should be considered for slowing cognitive decline. In a patient with prominent insomnia, psychosis, cardiovascular disease, or gastrointestinal problems, I would suggest memantine over cholinesterase inhibitors.

Other Medications

See Table 5–7 for a description of the use of medications that do not fall into any of the categories described. I have already discussed using acetaminophen; I recommend it be considered for every patient with BPSD without liver disease or active alcohol use.

Disturbances in noradrenergic functioning may contribute to BPSD. Accordingly, agents that act on the noradrenergic system have been studied. Propranolol augmentation of current psychotropic medication regimen provided modest short-term, but not sustained, improvement in agitation (Peskind et al. 2005). Prazosin was found to be effective for overall BPSD and well tolerated; see Table 5–7 for dosing (Wang et al. 2009). Unpublished results of a small, placebo-controlled study of prazosin 4 mg two times a day by the same group appear to be positive; the most common side effects of prazosin were sedation and dizziness (E.R. Peskind, "Prazosin Treatment for Disruptive Agitation in Alzheimer's Disease," May 21, 2015. Available at: https://clinicaltrials.gov/ct2/show/results/NCT01126099). A trial of prazosin would be reasonable in patients who have not responded to or tolerated antidepressants and antipsychotics.

See the next two sections for discussion of pimavanserin, dextromethorphan-quinidine, and stimulants.

INTERVENTIONS BY SYMPTOM

Thus far, I have been referring to the treatment of BPSD in the aggregate and agitation in particular. I now move on to other symptom-specific interventions.

Depression, Anxiety, Irritability, Emotional Lability, and Suicidality

In general, studies of antidepressants (including sertraline, citalopram, escitalopram, and mirtazapine) specifically for depression (as opposed to agitation or overall BPSD) in dementia have had disappointing results; anxiety has been less well studied, and so far trials have been negative (Farina et al. 2017). There are no controlled trials of the anxiolytic buspirone in persons with dementia. Nonpharmacological approaches are more promising: as noted, individual psychotherapy may be effective for patients with depression and less severe dementia, and exercise may be of benefit. Table 5–2 includes guidance for family caregivers under "Responding to depression and anxiety."

Dextromethorphan, combined with quinidine to prolong the half-life of dextromethorphan and allow for twice-daily dosing, has been found to be effective at reducing pseudobulbar affect (also known as pathological laughing and crying). Dextromethorphan-quinidine is also effective in patients with dementia due to AD, decreasing agitation, irritability, lability, depression, and overall BPSD (Cummings et al. 2015); it is a reasonable choice for patients who have not responded to or tolerated antidepressants and antipsychotics. See Table 5–7 for dosing and precautions.

Early dementia and a recent diagnosis of dementia are risk factors for suicide, and psychosocial interventions may reduce suicidal ideation (Kiosses et al. 2015). There are no studies of pharmacological interventions specifically for suicidal ideation in dementia.

Electroconvulsive therapy (ECT) appears to be effective for depression in dementia but is associated with delirium (in the Oudman (2012) study, affecting half of patients with dementia and depression who received ECT), falls, hip fracture, pneumonia, and a 30-day mortality rate of 6% (Kaster and Blumberger 2018; Oudman 2012). Interestingly, ECT has also been found to be effective for agitation and aggression in dementia (van den Berg et al. 2018). Personally, I think that the difficulty obtaining consent for ECT from a patient with dementia and agitation and the logistical difficulties of administering ECT to an agitated patient make ECT an impractical option for agitation.

Hallucinations and Delusions

Some of the literature cited thus far has already covered treatment of psychosis; also, I cover psychosis associated with Lewy body disease in greater detail later in "Special Considerations by Diagnosis." Hallucinations and delusions in and of themselves do not necessarily warrant treatment with antipsychotics or other medications. Some hallucinations may be benign or not troubling. Some delusions may not be particularly intense, and distraction might be a suitable intervention. In most cases, I recommend caregiver education on how best to respond (see Table 5–2). In the case of auditory or visual hallucinations, the clinician should ensure that hearing and vision loss have been addressed, as discussed earlier. I recommend pharmacologically addressing hallucinations or delusions only if they are distressing to the patient and nonpharmacological interventions have failed, or if they are spurring on behavior that is dangerous to the patient or others (e.g., paranoid ideation leading to physical aggression directed toward caregivers). It should be noted that antipsychotics appear to be less effective for psychosis than for agitation.

A trial of pimavanserin for psychosis associated with AD found benefit after 6 weeks but not after 12 weeks (Ballard et al. 2018). I would consider pimavanserin only for patients with Lewy body disease, discussed in greater detail later.

Sexual Aggression

Sexuality is a core part of the human experience, and interest in sex may continue well into late life. However, when combined with diminished frontal lobe function (and hence impulse control), interest in sex may result in unwanted or problematic behavior, including inappropriate sexual language and sexual acts (touching or grabbing others, exposing oneself, requesting unnecessary genital care, or masturbating in public) (De Giorgi and Series 2016). Environmental interventions in residential settings can include moving patients to single rooms, making provisions for conjugal visits, changing the gender of caregivers, and avoiding overstimulating television programs; behavioral interventions include redirection, distraction, and increased activities; and psychoeducation of family and caregivers may be helpful (De Giorgi and Series 2016). There are no RCTs of medications for sexual behaviors, but there are reports of benefit with SSRIs, trazodone, antipsychotics, anticonvulsants (specifically, carbamazepine and gabapentin), and hormonal therapies (medroxyprogesterone, finasteride, oral or transdermal estrogen, and leuprolide) (De Giorgi and Series 2016).

Wandering

Table 5–2 lists suggested nonpharmacological strategies to reduce the risks associated with a person with dementia wandering away from home. Electronic tagging of patients at risk of wandering in a hospital or residential setting may be effective (Cipriani et al. 2014). Risperidone 1 mg/day can decrease wandering; there are otherwise very few studies of medications for wandering (Cipriani et al. 2014). In the United States, the Alzheimer's Association offers the MedicAlert+Safe Return program, which provides an identification bracelet for the person with dementia to wear and a 24-hour service for reporting missing persons with dementia.

Disturbances of Sleep

A Cochrane review of pharmacological interventions for sleep disturbance in dementia found that trazodone 50 mg at bedtime was well tolerated and improved sleep (McCleery et al. 2016). Multiple studies of melatonin (up to 10 mg/day for 8–10 weeks) failed to demonstrate efficacy, and the melatonin agonist ramelteon was also ineffective. The authors found no RCTs of benzodiazepines or nonbenzodiazepine hypnotics (McCleery et al. 2016). A small study of mirtazapine 15 mg at bedtime for 2 weeks found that it did not improve insomnia but did increase daytime sleepiness (Scoralick et al. 2017).

Light therapy is not effective for BPSD in general or sleep disturbance in particular. A behavioral program involving sleep hygiene education, daily walking, and increased light exposure over the course of 2 months found sustained improvement for up to 6 months (McCurry et al. 2005). Family caregivers may find the tips in Table 5–2 useful.

REM sleep behavior disorder, which is associated with Lewy body disease, can be distressing to caregivers and dangerous to patients and bed partners. Clonazepam is first-line treatment for REM sleep behavior disorder, with some evidence that melatonin may be helpful. For patients with sleep apnea and dementia, the long-term use of continuous positive airway pressure (CPAP) improved both cognition and mood (Cooke et al. 2009). There are no clinical trials of medications for restless legs syndrome in dementia, despite its potential contribution to nocturnal agitation; note that psychotropic medications can cause or exacerbate this condition.

In summary, except for trazodone for insomnia and clonazepam or melatonin for REM sleep behavior disorder, it does not appear that pharmacological interventions are helpful for sleep disorders. I would generally recommend a behavioral approach instead.

Apathy

Despite how prevalent and persistent apathy is across the course of dementia (van der Linde et al. 2016) and how frustrating apathy is to family members in my clinical practice, very minimal literature exists on reducing apathy.

Methylphenidate may be helpful for patients with apathy due to AD (Ruthi-rakuhan et al. 2018) but is associated with hypertension—specifically, an 18-mmHg increase in blood pressure with 10 mg twice a day (Padala et al. 2018). No other medications have been found to be helpful for apathy in AD (Ruthirakuhan et al. 2018). Music therapy, multisensory interventions, and perhaps pet therapy can reduce apathy (Scales et al. 2018). See the subsection "Frontotemporal Dementia" for discussion of the use of stimulants in FTD.

Anorexia and Weight Loss

Weight loss is common in patients with dementia. Medications that can reduce appetite (which could include cholinesterase inhibitors) should be discontinued, and nausea, abdominal pain, and constipation should be addressed. Nonpharmacological interventions include high-calorie dietary supplements, increasing protein intake, and daily physical activity (Droogsma et al. 2015). A small retrospective study found that mirtazapine 30 mg/day was associated with a weight gain of 1.9 kg (4 lbs) over 3 months and 2.1 kg (4.6 lbs) at 6 months; patients with lower BMI at baseline gained more weight (Segers and Surquin 2014). Note that lower dosages (7.5–15 mg/day) of mirtazapine are more likely to stimulate appetite than higher dosages (30–45 mg/day). Feeding tubes are associated with worse outcomes and should not be placed (Palecek et al. 2010).

Elation and Mania

The evidence base supporting the use of lithium and atypical antipsychotics in late-life bipolar disorder is limited. I am not aware of any pharmacological or nonpharmacological studies for elation or mania specifically in patients with dementia.

SPECIAL CONSIDERATIONS BY DIAGNOSIS

Most of the literature reviewed above pertains to patients with AD. However, a significant number of patients with BPSD, including those treated with antipsychotics, do not have AD. Table 5–8 summarizes what is known about how treatment differs in persons with other causes of dementia, as described in greater detail in this section.

Lewy Body Disease

One of the most common psychiatric manifestations of DLB and PDD is visual hallucinations, which in other contexts would be treated with anti-

TABLE 5–8. Special considerations in treating behavioral and psychological symptoms of non-Alzheimer's causes of dementia

Cause of dementia	Most common behavioral and psychological symptoms	Treatment considerations
Lewy body disease, namely, either DLB or PDD	Visual hallucinations, delusions, anxiety, sleep disturbance due to REM sleep behavior disorder, fluctuations of symptoms that may resemble delirium or sundowning	Donepezil should be first-line treatment. Patients are very sensitive to the side effects of antipsychotics—specifically, more prone to EPS and higher risk of mortality. If an antipsychotic is to be used, consider quetiapine and clozapine over risperidone and aripiprazole. Levodopa, used to treat motor symptoms, may cause or exacerbate psychosis.
Vascular dementia	Apathy, amotivation, depression	Patients may be at higher risk of stroke or cardiac complications of antipsychotics. Consider a stimulant for apathy, but monitor for cardiovascular and cerebrovascular complications.
FTD, behavioral variant	Disinhibition, verbal repetitiveness, verbal aggression, physical aggression, hyperorality, apathy	Behavioral disturbances can be severe and dangerous. Consider trazodone and SSRIs as first-line agents. A stimulant could be used with caution, monitoring for worsening symptoms. Avoid cholinesterase inhibitors and memantine. Very little literature on antipsychotics.
Intellectual or developmental disability, including Down syndrome	Depression, apathy, compulsions	Donepezil may help with cognitive impairment; use low doses to improve tolerability. SSRIs may aid compulsions. Use all other psychotropic medications with caution.

Note.   DLB=dementia with Lewy bodies; EPS=extrapyramidal symptoms; FTD=frontotemporal dementia; PDD=Parkinson disease dementia; REM=rapid eye movement; SSRIs=selective serotonin reuptake inhibitors.

psychotic medications. However, patients with DLB and PDD are especially prone to side effects from antipsychotics, including EPS and death (Reus et al. 2016). Therefore, the caution regarding the use of antipsychotics in patients in dementia is even stronger when the underlying pathology is Lewy body disease.

Instead, cholinesterase inhibitors should be prescribed. A meta-analysis of eight controlled trials of donepezil or rivastigmine for DLB or PDD demonstrated improved global outcomes; BPSD were improved in subjects with PDD but not in those with DLB (Stinton et al. 2015). One uncontrolled trial found that donepezil may be useful specifically for reducing visual hallucinations (Satoh et al. 2010). The most commonly reported side effects of cholinesterase inhibitors used in DLB or PDD are nausea, vomiting, anorexia, tremor, somnolence, dizziness, and insomnia; donepezil appears to be better tolerated than rivastigmine (Stinton et al. 2015). The patch formulation of rivastigmine has fewer gastrointestinal side effects than the oral formulation and could be used when a person with dementia has difficulty swallowing. Sudden withdrawal of donepezil may result in a marked increase in BPSD and worsening of cognition (Minett et al. 2003). There is less evidence supporting the use of galantamine than either donepezil or rivastigmine (Stinton et al. 2015). Therefore, I recommend donepezil as a first-line treatment (more tolerable than rivastigmine), rivastigmine second (more data on efficacy than galantamine), and galantamine third within this class.

Levodopa, used to ameliorate motor symptoms of DLB or PDD, can exacerbate psychosis (Stinton et al. 2015). The dopamine agonist pramipexole is modestly effective for depression in patients with Parkinson disease, but dopamine agonists have not been studied in patients with dementia and can cause hallucinations (Connolly and Lang 2014). Careful coordination between a patient's neurologist and other treatment providers is necessary to balance the medications used to address motor symptoms and the medications used to address BPSD. In fact, for a patient with DLB or PDD and psychosis, consideration should be given to decreasing or discontinuing antiparkinsonian treatments prior to starting a new medication (Connolly and Lang 2014).

Very limited evidence (mostly in the form of case series) suggests possible efficacy for duloxetine (depression), escitalopram (depression), trazodone (depression), clonazepam (sleep disturbance), ramelteon (sleep disturbance), gabapentin (agitation, restless legs), and zonisamide (overall BPSD) (Stinton et al. 2015). Memantine and citalopram have not been found to be effective for BPSD in patients with DLB or PDD (Stinton et al. 2015).

Do atypical antipsychotics have a role in treating BPSD in patients with Lewy body disease, especially those with hallucinations or delusions? In situations where psychosis is especially distressing to patients or leading to dangerous behaviors, an antipsychotic could be considered. On the basis of studies of psychosis in Parkinson disease, clozapine has the strongest evidence for efficacy, whereas the evidence supporting quetiapine is generally not encouraging (four negative RCTs and one positive RCT) (Connolly and Lang 2014). Clozapine and quetiapine are less likely to exacerbate the motor symptoms of DLB or PDD than are risperidone, aripiprazole, and olanzapine. Clozapine can result in agranulocytosis and therefore requires monitoring of absolute neutrophil count and, in many countries, registration of the patient with a national registry; in fact, it appears that the risk of agranulocytosis is higher in older adults than in younger adults (Bishara and Taylor 2014). Other important side effects of clozapine include sedation, weight gain, new-onset diabetes mellitus or dyslipidemia, anticholinergic effects, myocarditis, cardiomyopathy, orthostatic hypotension, sialorrhea, seizures, and urinary incontinence (Bishara and Taylor 2014). Therefore, quetiapine is typically prescribed before clozapine. I recommend using olanzapine only with extreme caution and at low dosages (2.5–5 mg/day), and I advise against using risperidone, aripiprazole, and any typical antipsychotic.

Pimavanserin was recently approved in the United States for the treatment of Parkinson disease psychosis (Table 5–7). This medication is a selective serotonin 5-HT$_{2A}$ inverse agonist and does not have any dopaminergic activity. Its evidence for efficacy in Parkinson disease psychosis is modest, and it can cause QT prolongation as well as drug-drug interactions (Bozymski et al. 2017). Additionally, the FDA has raised concern about an increased risk of mortality associated with pimavanserin. The high cost and the need to use a specialty pharmacy limit the use of pimavanserin (Bozymski et al. 2017).

Vascular Dementia

There is a robust literature regarding the treatment of poststroke depression and other psychiatric sequelae, but it is not clear how applicable the findings are to most patients with vascular dementia and associated BPSD. One uncontrolled trial of antipsychotics specifically for patients with vascular dementia and BPSD found that olanzapine and haloperidol were equally effective at reducing symptoms (Moretti et al. 2005). Many trials of antipsychotics for BPSD in AD also enrolled subjects with vascular dementia or mixed (Alzheimer's and vascular) dementia; therefore, perhaps the evidence regarding safety and efficacy of antipsychotics detailed earlier also applies to patients with vascular dementia (see Reus et al. [2016] for a detailed list of antipsychotic trials that included subjects with vascular dementia or mixed dementia). Presumably, patients with vascular dementia have vascular risk factors that put them at higher risk of cardiovascular morbidity and mortality relative to other causes of dementia; however, a retrospective study found that patients with vascular dementia treated with antipsychotics (specifically, risperidone or quetiapine) did not have a higher risk of death than those not prescribed antipsychotics (Sultana et al. 2014).

Stimulants may be useful for apathy and excess daytime sedation in vascular dementia but can cause significant side effects, including hypertension, tachycardia, irritability, and agitation (Dolder et al. 2010). Hypertension and tachycardia are especially concerning given patients' risk for cerebrovascular and cardiovascular events.

One uncontrolled trial of galantamine in patients with AD with or without vascular dementia found improvements in anxiety, delusions, and diurnal rhythm disturbances (Tangwongchai et al. 2008).

There is mixed evidence regarding the efficacy of group reminiscence therapy for patients with vascular dementia (Akanuma et al. 2011; Ito et al. 2007). Otherwise, there do not appear to be any studies of nonpharmacological interventions specifically for BPSD in patients with vascular dementia.

Frontotemporal Dementia

The behaviors of a person with FTD—including disinhibition, hyperorality, and apathy—can be particularly distressing to caregivers and potentially unsafe for patients and caregivers (Nardell and Tampi 2014). Patients with FTD are relatively young and therefore may be physically healthy and even vigorous, making the management of symptoms even more challenging.

The limited literature on treating the behavioral symptoms of FTD suggests that serotonergic agents, including SSRIs and trazodone, may be helpful (Herrmann et al. 2012; Nardell and Tampi 2014). Studies of SSRIs have involved paroxetine and citalopram, but paroxetine should probably be avoided because of associated cognitive impairment, presumably due to anticholinergic properties (Nardell and Tampi 2014). For citalopram, the dosage range in an open-label study was 10–40 mg/day, with the 40-mg/day dosage associated with higher risk of side effects, including agitation; QT prolongation may be an issue at dosages above 20 mg/day (Herrmann et al. 2012). Trazodone 150–300 mg/day was effective at reducing BPSD in FTD, with the most common side effects being fatigue, dizziness, hypotension, and cold extremities (Nardell and Tampi 2014). I would recommend dividing trazodone into two or three doses per day: a larger bedtime dose to aid with insomnia and one or two smaller daytime doses to aid with daytime agitation (daytime dosing can be associated with sedation and falls).

The only controlled study of an antipsychotic in FTD (using quetiapine 150 mg/day) was negative (Nardell and Tampi 2014); another study suggested that patients with FTD have heightened sensitivity to the side effects of antipsychotics (Reus et al. 2016). Nevertheless, I suspect that antipsychotics are often prescribed because of the severe nature of BPSD in patients with FTD. The risk of mortality associated with antipsychotics in FTD is unknown; it would be prudent to consider the risk to be the same as in AD when informing patients and their proxy decision makers of the risks of antipsychotics.

Stimulant trials have been promising. Methylphenidate 40 mg/day may help address disinhibition, and dextroamphetamine 20 mg/day may help with both disinhibition and apathy; hypertension is a concern when using stimulants (Nardell and Tampi 2014). There are case reports of topiramate being effective for abnormal eating behavior in FTD, and there are case reports of bupropion being effective for apathy.

Given the efficacy of dextromethorphan-quinidine for pseudobulbar affect, this treatment would be reasonable to consider for patients with FTD. Thus far, no controlled trials have been reported; there is one case report, indicating improvement in behavioral symptoms in a patient with FTD treated with dextromethorphan-quinidine (Chen et al. 2018).

Cholinesterase inhibitors and memantine are best avoided, because there is some evidence that they may worsen cognition or cause agitation in patients with FTD (Young et al. 2018). There do not appear to be any trials of nonpharmacological interventions specifically for patients with FTD.

Intellectual or Developmental Disability

By age 40 years, almost all people with Down syndrome will have neuropathological changes consistent with AD; by age 60, about half will have clinical evidence of dementia (Moran et al. 2013). The National Task Group on Intellectual Disabilities and Dementia Practice has developed a tool for screening for dementia in persons with intellectual and developmental disability (I/DD), available online (http://aadmd.org/ntg/screening). Nevertheless, the literature on treating BPSD in persons with I/DD in general and Down syndrome in particular is very limited (Moran et al. 2013). Donepezil may be effective for cognitive symptoms in Down syndrome but was also associated with more side effects than expected; it has been recommended that the starting and target dosages of donepezil be lower than usual (Hefti and Blanco 2017). There is very modest evidence that SSRIs can reduce compulsions (Hefti and Blanco 2017). Memantine does not appear to be helpful (Moran et al. 2013). In general, I am concerned about the tolerability of psychotropic medications in persons with I/DD, and I recommend emphasizing nonpharmacological approaches.

SPECIAL CONSIDERATIONS BY SETTING

Though most of the principles of management described in this chapter may apply to most settings in which a patient with dementia may be, there are unique aspects to managing BPSD in patients at home; in an LTC facility; in an emergency department; in an inpatient medical, surgical, or psychiatric unit; in a palliative care or hospice setting; or in a jail or prison.

Patient or Family Home

Most people with dementia live in their own homes and do not have formal (paid) caregivers; however, most studies of interventions for BPSD have not been conducted with subjects who still live at home. As noted earlier in this chapter, educational interventions for family caregivers have had mixed evidence, although attending support groups may be helpful. A home-based intervention wherein occupational therapists, over the course of eight sessions, train family caregivers of veterans how to implement structured activities tailored to the capabilities and interests of the person with dementia has been shown to be effective (Gitlin et al. 2018).

Clinicians should also encourage family caregivers to hire formal caregivers or others who can help with housework, to consider having the person with dementia participate in adult day care, and to obtain respite care. Table 5–2 lists other specific advice for family caregivers.

Clinicians may find it useful to structure their interventions with family caregivers around nonpharmacological goals they can accomplish with their loved ones. During a clinic visit, the clinician can work collaboratively to determine progress made on prior goals and to set new goals as needed. See Figure 5–2 for a worksheet that aids this process.

Long-Term Care Facility

Given that approximately 60% of residents of LTC facilities have dementia and that BPSD are a common reason for admission from home to LTC settings, the prevalence of BPSD would be expected to be high in LTC settings (Seitz et al. 2012). Many studies of nonpharmacological interventions for BPSD have been conducted in LTC settings, so much of the discussion of nonpharmacological interventions is germane here. There is evidence of

PLAN OF CARE

Patient's name: _____   Today's date: ___ / ___ / _____

QUALITY OF LIFE
What is most important to the patient now? What does she or he enjoy doing?

GOAL DISCUSSED AT THIS VISIT
Be as **specific** as possible, and make sure that the goal is **measurable**, **achievable**, **relevant**, and to be accomplished in a certain amount of **time**.

INTERVENTION(S)
What will help you accomplish this goal?

    1.
    2.
    3.

MEASURING CHANGE
How will we know if the patient is meeting the goal?

RESOURCES AND OTHER RECOMMENDATIONS

FIGURE 5–2.   Behavioral management worksheet for use with family care-givers.

During an office visit, a clinician can work together with the patient and family caregiver to develop a SMART goal (see Table 5–3) and plan of care. A SMART goal is specific, measurable, achievable, relevant, and accomplishable in a certain amount of time.

Source.   © 2018, Eileen Ahearn, M.D., Ph.D. Used with permission.

modest efficacy for training LTC staff, increasing patient activities, music therapy, aromatherapy, and geriatric mental health consultation programs (Seitz et al. 2012). There have been no comparisons of pharmacological and nonpharmacological interventions for BPSD in LTC settings (Seitz et al. 2012).

The Alzheimer's Association (2009) recommends that the staff of assisted living facilities and nursing homes receive initial and ongoing training in the following topics:

- Dementia, including memory loss and progression of cognitive impairment
- Behavioral and psychological symptoms of dementia, as well as understanding and addressing these symptoms
- Strategies for providing person-centered care
- Communicating effectively with residents with dementia
- Family dynamics
- Addressing pain
- Ensuring that residents have adequate hydration and nutrition
- Promoting residents' social engagement

Staff will also need their own emotional support as they deal with challenging behaviors and witness a resident's decline and death (Alzheimer's Association 2009).

Dementia care mapping has been recommended to improve the quality of care provided to residents with dementia in LTC settings; it has some evidence for efficacy in reducing BPSD among residents and burnout among staff (Surr et al. 2018). A specially trained "mapper" investigates the care processes in place in an LTC facility and then provides feedback for improvement plans to be applied at a resident-specific level and at the institutional level. It appears that this approach works best in facilities that have adopted a person-centered approach as opposed to facilities that have yet to make this cultural shift (Surr et al. 2018).

In the United States, federal regulations govern the use of psychotropic medications among residents of LTC facilities. The nursing home reform provisions of the Omnibus Budget Reconciliation Act of 1987, which restricts the use of antipsychotics among LTC residents and requires attempts at gradual dose reduction of antipsychotics, resulted in decreased prescription of antipsychotics to LTC residents (Bharani and Snowden 2005).

Nevertheless, antipsychotics are the most studied pharmacological intervention for LTC residents with BPSD, and, consistent with other studies, the evidence of efficacy is generally modest (Bharani and Snowden 2005). There is some evidence of efficacy for citalopram and carbamazepine (Bharani and Snowden 2005).

Emergency Department

Patients with severe BPSD might be taken to an emergency department for evaluation and management. Bessey et al. (2018) detailed how to care for older adults with behavioral health emergencies, including agitation and psychosis, in the emergency department. (All of the information in this section is drawn from their review.) The patient's cognitive impairment and agitation may make it difficult to collect a full history of symptoms and recent events. The department staff may need to contact family members, the staff of the patient's residence, other caregivers, or health care providers to obtain the history. Delirium should be considered the most likely etiology of agitation or psychosis, and a medical workup should be pursued accordingly. Causes of pain should be carefully considered, including problems with dentition, constipation, urinary retention, and skin ulceration. The clinician should order diagnostic testing necessary to rule in or out suspected etiologies of BPSD.

As in other settings, nonpharmacological treatment is preferred to pharmacological treatment. Nonpharmacological options that can be used in the emergency department include the following:

- Warm or weighted blanket
- Addressing the patient at his or her eye level
- Providing nourishment
- Using a calm voice with short, simple phrases
- Validating frustration and fear
- Keeping the number of people in the patient's room to a minimum
- Ensuring that the patient has access to assistive devices, such as hearing aids and glasses
- Reorienting the patient
- Providing a one-to-one sitter
- Asking family members or other caregivers to help reassure and calm the patient

If the patient's behavior poses a risk to self or to the treatment team, a medication may be indicated. Oral antipsychotics, at the lowest dosage necessary to be effective, are considered first-line treatment but should be avoided in patients with DLB and PDD. Benzodiazepines should be avoided unless alcohol withdrawal is thought to be the cause of BPSD. There are case reports of death in patients given a combination of parenteral olanzapine and benzodiazepine. Physical restraints should not be used except in situations of extreme danger to the patient or others.

Inpatient Medical, Surgical, or Psychiatric Unit

The presence of BPSD increases patients' risk of admission to inpatient units, both psychiatric and nonpsychiatric, and BPSD are common among patients with dementia who are hospitalized; unfortunately, hospital staff may not be adequately trained in the management of BPSD and may find that dealing with these situations contributes to burnout (Gitlin et al. 2016). One implication of this is that measures should be taken at home to reduce risk factors for hospital admission—for example, by addressing BPSD prior to their becoming severe enough to warrant hospitalization (Toot et al. 2013). Nursing guidelines for how to respond to BPSD on inpatient medical/surgical units echo the recommended behavioral and communication approaches described in the "Emergency Department" subsection (e.g., be reassuring, avoid arguing, use distraction or redirection, maintain a routine, minimize noise and distractions). In addition, the guidelines recommend the following (Sparks 2008):

- Having a knowledgeable family member or friend stay with the patient during the hospitalization
- Avoiding the use of restraints
- Encouraging that familiar objects be brought from home
- Maintaining a warm room temperature and keeping the patient covered
- Maintaining usual and desired religious or spiritual practices
- Using specific techniques to aid with eating and drinking
- Camouflaging tubes and dressing to decrease the chance that the patient will try to remove them
- Placing inpatients at risk for wandering in a room that is easy for staff to monitor
- Scheduling toileting upon waking, before meals, at bedtime, after fluid intake, and after diuretic administration
- Minimizing the distress associated with bathing—for example, using a shower with a handheld showerhead, a tub bath, or a sponge bath

There are a number of small studies of nonpharmacological interventions on inpatient psychiatric units. For example, the Tailored Activity Program (TAP) is an intervention that has been found to be feasible (though efficacy is as yet unknown) in an inpatient psychiatric setting: staff identify the interests and capabilities of each person with dementia and in turn develop a plan to tailor activities and train families to do the same after discharge (Gitlin et al. 2016). Two studies found that multisensory stimulation on inpatient psychiatric units, including Snoezelen, are effective (Brasure et al. 2016). Although state psychiatric hospitals may be sites of care of patients with severe BPSD, I am not aware of any specific literature in that setting.

Palliative Care and Hospice

Many aspects of the palliative care approach are consonant with the approach detailed in this chapter, including the focus on promoting quality of life, close attention to managing pain, and withdrawal of unnecessary medications. Medications to consider discontinuing in patients with advanced dementia include cognitive enhancers, lipid-lowering agents, vitamin supplements, antiplatelet agents, hormones, cytotoxic chemotherapy agents, and leukotriene inhibitors; antipsychotics and antidepressants may be appropriate, based on careful review of risks and benefits (Lee et al. 2018). The approach to pain management differs somewhat, given the greater acceptance of use of opioids. A person with dementia can qualify for hospice care when life expectancy is 6 months or less (typically, Functional Assessment Staging [FAST] stage 7, plus one or more conditions indicating that one is approaching end of life, such as weight loss >10% over the past 6 months); beginning hospice care will bring additional resources to the patient and caregivers that may reduce caregiver burden (Lee et al. 2018). My own experience is that many patients and family caregivers are either unaware of or do not take advantage of palliative care or hospice services, and I recommend that clinicians bring up these services with patients and families at least once.

Jail or Prison

The incarcerated population, like the rest of the population, is aging. Although the prevalence of dementia in prison is unclear (estimates range from 1% to 44% of older prisoners), it is estimated that the number of prisoners with dementia will double by 2030 and triple by 2050; however, only 4% of U.S. prisons offer geriatric-specific health care services. The content in this section is drawn from the review by Maschi et al. (2012).

Dementia may interfere with a prisoner's ability to follow prison rules and protocols, and behavioral symptoms can be misconstrued as volitional; in these situations, patients may be exposed to punishment (e.g., solitary confinement) that could exacerbate BPSD. Furthermore, prisoners with dementia may be at increased risk of being victimized physically or sexually. The following recommendations have been suggested to address BPSD in correctional settings:

- Training staff to detect dementia, to identify BPSD, and to communicate in an empathic and respectful way
- Providing protective housing to create a dementia-friendly environment or making modifications to the environment to reduce stress
- Increasing physical or health-promoting activities
- Offering group activities involving, for example, art, pet therapy, music, and peer support

SPECIAL CONSIDERATIONS IN MINORITY POPULATIONS

In the section "Cultural and Spiritual Factors" in Chapter 4, I reviewed cultural considerations in the assessment of patients with BPSD. I now turn to treatment. Ethnic minority elders face barriers to care, resulting in delays in receiving appropriate dementia care (Cooper et al. 2010). African Americans are less likely to be prescribed cognitive enhancers than are white patients, and African Americans prescribed cholinesterase inhibitors are less likely than whites to be continuing to take them 6 months later (Cooper et al. 2010).

There is evidence that caregiver interventions may need to be tailored based on the caregiver's ethnic background. Dementia caregivers vary in their response to BPSD by ethnicity. For example, fewer Hispanic caregivers expressed confidence in responding to verbal aggression than did African American and white caregivers, suggesting that caregivers need tailored interventions (Hansen et al. 2018). An in-home respite program and adult day care in the United States tailored to the needs of ethnic minority (specifically, African American and Hispanic) elders found *greater* utilization by these ethnic minority elders than by white elders (Cooper et al. 2010). A large multicenter trial for an intervention for family caregivers that intentionally included African American and Hispanic subjects has been found to be effective; the intervention comprised 12 in-home and telephone sessions addressing caregiver depression, burden, self-care, social support, and responding to BPSD (Belle et al. 2006). An in-home behavioral management program, a psychoeducation skills training program, and an individualized counseling and support program, all tailored to Chinese cultural values, were found to be helpful in reducing distress among Chinese American caregivers (Sun et al. 2012). A cognitive-behavioral therapy group intervention for Latino caregivers resulted in both less caregiver distress and a reduction in BPSD (Gonyea et al. 2016).

I looked for literature regarding specific considerations for ethnic minority elders receiving psychopharmacological treatment for BPSD. I found only a report that African American elders exposed to antipsychotics are more likely than others to develop tardive dyskinesia (Woerner et al. 2011).

Lesbian, gay, bisexual, transgender, and queer (LGBTQ) elders and their partners have reported being refused social services after identifying their gender identity or sexuality, which may lead to delays in care and inadequate support (Barrett et al. 2015). Dementia may lead to LGBTQ elders being more vulnerable to homophobic or transphobic views within their family of origin, which in turn could lead to elder abuse (Barrett et al. 2015). Creating an environment of inclusivity is important in services for LGBTQ elders with dementia and in support groups for their caregivers (Barrett et al. 2015).

The literature on HIV dementia suggests that stimulants may be helpful for apathy and depression and that patients with HIV dementia may be more likely to develop EPS from antipsychotics. However, it is unclear how relevant this information is to the care of LGBTQ elders with other causes of dementia (and, of course, not all patients with HIV dementia are LGBTQ).

SUMMARY: SAFELY AND EFFECTIVELY CARING FOR A PERSON WITH BPSD

Understanding who the person with dementia is, what behavioral symptoms are of concern, and what the context is in which they are occurring is essential to developing a treatment plan for BPSD. The plan will typically include addressing underlying medical issues, eliminating medications and other substances that could be contributing to BPSD, educating and supporting the patient and caregiver, and nonpharmacological interventions (activity, stimulation, behavior management); and in some cases, pharmacological interventions are included. The specific BPSD and the underlying cause of dementia will help inform the treatment plan. All patients and their family members should be cared for in a respectful, compassionate, and culturally sensitive way.

KEY POINTS

- The initial step in managing BPSD is addressing any medical problems that have been identified as potential contributors to BPSD, including infection, electrolyte disturbance, constipation, urinary retention, and hearing and vision loss.
  - Untreated or undertreated pain is common in patients with dementia. Scheduling acetaminophen at dosages up to 3,000 mg/day can be a safe and effective intervention.
  - Clinicians should discontinue or reduce dosages of medications and other substances that could be causing or contributing to BPSD, especially medications with anticholinergic properties, sedative-hypnotic drugs, opioids, and alcohol.
- Resources to support and educate patients, family members, and other caregivers should be provided.
- Nonpharmacological interventions should be tried before pharmacological interventions.
  - Training of formal caregivers is overall the most effective intervention for BPSD. The staff of facilities caring for persons with dementia should be trained in patient-centered care, communication skills, and behavioral principles.
  - Other nonpharmacological interventions that may be of benefit include scheduling activities, music therapy, therapeutic touch or massage, and other sensory interventions.
  - Individual psychotherapy, specifically reminiscence therapy and problem-solving therapy, may be helpful for depression.
- Pharmacological interventions should be prescribed only when BPSD are potentially dangerous to the person with dementia or to caregivers or when BPSD cause significant distress to the person with dementia.
  - Antidepressants: Citalopram, escitalopram, and trazodone have the strongest evidence of efficacy, primarily for agitation rather than depression or anxiety.
  - Antipsychotics: Risperidone, olanzapine, and aripiprazole have the strongest evidence of efficacy, but the entire category has extensive side effects, including death.
  - Anticonvulsants: Carbamazepine has the best evidence for efficacy, but drug-drug interactions and side effects are problematic. Valproate should not be used. Gabapentin could be considered.

- Benzodiazepines: These medications should not be used except for emergency management of severe BPSD (lorazepam) or REM sleep behavior disorder (clonazepam).
- Cognitive enhancers: Cholinesterase inhibitors and memantine are unlikely to have much benefit for treatment of BPSD but can be prescribed to delay cognitive decline.
- Other: Dextromethorphan-quinidine and prazosin can be considered.

• Most of the literature on pharmacological interventions relates to agitation, psychosis, and overall BPSD. Effective treatments for other BPSD, including depression, are less clear.

• Disease-specific interventions include the following:

- Lewy body disease: Donepezil should be the first-line treatment for BPSD. Antipsychotics should be avoided—but, if deemed necessary, quetiapine or clozapine could be used. It is unclear what role pimavanserin will ultimately have.
- Vascular dementia: A stimulant may be helpful for apathy but comes with a risk of hypertension and tachycardia.
- FTD: Some evidence supports use of an SSRI, trazodone, or stimulant. Very limited data are available on antipsychotics.
- Intellectual or developmental disability: Donepezil may help cognitive impairment, and SSRIs may help compulsions. Data on other medications are very limited. Patients should be monitored closely for side effects.

• Ethnic minority elders face barriers to care, resulting in delays in receiving appropriate dementia care, including for BPSD. To be effective, caregiver interventions may need to be tailored based on a caregiver's ethnic background.

• LGBTQ persons with dementia and their caregivers may face discrimination when seeking care. Creating an environment of inclusivity is important in services for LGBTQ elders with dementia and in support groups for their caregivers.

RESOURCES FOR PATIENTS, FAMILIES, AND CAREGIVERS

AgingCare: Family Caring for Family. Naples, FL, AgingCare, 2017. Available at: www.agingcare.com/ebooks/family-caregiver?ebs=lib. This eBook goes well beyond managing BPSD to cover a wide range of topics related to being the caregiver for a person with dementia, including communicating with family members, the health care system, understanding options for senior housing, and taking care of oneself as a caregiver.

ALZConnected (www.alzconnected.org) is a free online community for people affected by dementia, including patients and their caregivers, and is hosted by the Alzheimer's Association.

Alzheimer's Association: Stages and Behaviors. Chicago, IL, Alzheimer's Association, 2018. Available at: https://www.alz.org/help-support/caregiving/stages-behaviors. This web page describes how caregivers can respond to behaviors. There are links to tips on a number of topics, including how to respond to agitation, depression, anxiety, hallucinations, wandering, and other safety concerns.

Alzheimer's Disease International Factsheets (www.alz.co.uk/ADI-publications; scroll down to "Factsheets") are among a range of free publications produced by Alzheimer's Disease International. A factsheet on dementia and intellectual disabilities is available in English, Spanish, German, Chinese, Japanese, and Hebrew.

National Down Syndrome Society: Aging and Down Syndrome: A Health and Well-Being Guidebook. New York, National Down Syndrome Society, 2017. Available at: www.ndss.org/wp-content/uploads/2017/11/Aging-and-Down-Syndrome.pdf. The goal of this booklet is to provide guidance, education, and support to families and caregivers of older adults with Down syndrome; it includes specific suggestions to caregivers regarding the care of persons with Down syndrome who have developed AD.

National Institute on Aging: Caring for a Person With Alzheimer's Disease: Your Easy-to-Use Guide. Bethesda, MD, National Institute on Aging, 2017. Available at: https://order.nia.nih.gov/publication/caring-for-a-person-with-alzheimers-disease-your-easy-to-use-guide. This comprehensive and very readable guide includes extensive information for caregivers about why BPSD arise and how to address them. A PDF version can be downloaded, or up to 25 paper copies can be ordered; both options are free. Available in Spanish and English.

Spencer B, White L: Coping With Behavior Change in Dementia: A Family Caregiver's Guide. Ann Arbor, MI, Whisppub, 2015. This handbook is intended to help families understand possible causes of common behavior changes and learn to respond more effectively to dementia behaviors that care partners find challenging, including repetitive actions, agitation, and incontinence. The book also covers communication and problem solving and includes a glossary and an extensive list of books, videos, and other resources for people with dementia, family caregivers, and health care professionals. The authors maintain a blog at https://dementiacarebooks.com/ blogs.

REFERENCES

Abraha I, Rimland JM, Lozano-Montoya I, et al: Simulated presence therapy for dementia. Cochrane Database Syst Rev 4:CD011882, 2017 28418586

Akanuma K, Meguro K, Meguro M, et al: Improved social interaction and increased anterior cingulate metabolism after group reminiscence with reality orientation approach for vascular dementia. Psychiatry Res 192(3):183–187, 2011 21543189

Alzheimer's Association: Dementia Care Practice Recommendations for Assisted Living Residences and Nursing Homes. Chicago, IL, Alzheimer's Association, 2009. Available at: https://www.alz.org/national/documents/brochure_DCPRphases1n2.pdf. Accessed July 16, 2018.

Alzheimer's Association: Caregiving: Stages and Behaviors (website). Chicago, IL, Alzheimer's Association, 2018. Available at: https://www.alz.org/help-support/caregiving/stages-behaviors. Accessed July 15, 2018.

American Geriatrics Society 2019 Beers Criteria Update Expert Panel: American Geriatrics Society 2019 updated Beers Criteria for Potentially Inappropriate Medication Use in Older Adults. J Am Geriatr Soc 67(4):674–694, 2019 30693946

Ballard C, Hanney ML, Theodoulou M, et al: The dementia antipsychotic withdrawal trial (DART-AD): long-term follow-up of a randomised placebo-controlled trial. Lancet Neurol 8(2):151–157, 2009 19138567

Ballard C, Thomas A, Gerry S, et al: A double-blind randomized placebo-controlled withdrawal trial comparing memantine and antipsychotics for the long-term treatment of function and neuropsychiatric symptoms in people with Alzheimer's disease (MAIN-AD). J Am Med Dir Assoc 16(4):316–322, 2015 25523285

Ballard C, Banister C, Khan Z, et al: Evaluation of the safety, tolerability, and efficacy of pimavanserin versus placebo in patients with Alzheimer's disease psychosis: a phase 2, randomised, placebo-controlled, double-blind study. Lancet Neurol 17(3):213–222, 2018 29452684

Barreto PdeS, Demougeot L, Pillard F, et al: Exercise training for managing behavioral and psychological symptoms in people with dementia: a systematic review and meta-analysis. Ageing Res Rev 24(Pt B):274–285, 2015 26369357

Barrett C, Crameri P, Lambourne S, et al: Understanding the experiences and needs of lesbian, gay, bisexual and trans Australians living with dementia, and their partners. Australas J Ageing 34 (Suppl 2):34–38, 2005 26525445

Barry HE, Cooper JA, Ryan C, et al: Potentially inappropriate prescribing among people with dementia in primary care: a retrospective cross-sectional study using the enhanced prescribing database. J Alzheimers Dis 52(4):1503–1513, 2016 27079714

Belle SH, Burgio L, Burns R, et al: Enhancing the quality of life of dementia caregivers from different ethnic or racial groups: a randomized, controlled trial. Ann Intern Med 145(10):727–738, 2006 17116917

Bergh S, Selbæk G, Engedal K: Discontinuation of antidepressants in people with dementia and neuropsychiatric symptoms (DESEP study): double blind, randomised, parallel group, placebo controlled trial. BMJ 344:e1566, 2012 22408266

Bessey LJ, Radue RM, Chapman EN, et al: Behavioral health needs of older adults in the emergency department. Clin Geriatr Med 34(3):469–489, 2018 30031428

Bharani N, Snowden M: Evidence-based interventions for nursing home residents with dementia-related behavioral symptoms. Psychiatr Clin North Am 28(4):985–1005, x, 2005 16325737

Birkenhäger-Gillesse EG, Kollen BJ, Achterberg WP, et al: Effects of psychosocial interventions for behavioral and psychological symptoms in dementia on the prescription of psychotropic drugs: a systematic review and meta-analyses. J Am Med Dir Assoc 19(3):276.e1–276.e9, 2018 29477773

Bishara D, Taylor D: Adverse effects of clozapine in older patients: epidemiology, prevention and management. Drugs Aging 31(1):11–20, 2014 24338220

Bozymski KM, Lowe DK, Pasternak KM, et al: Pimavanserin: a novel antipsychotic for Parkinson's disease psychosis. Ann Pharmacother 51(6):479–487, 2017 28375643

Brasure M, Jutkowitz E, Fuchs E, et al: Nonpharmacologic Interventions for Agitation and Aggression in Dementia. Comparative Effectiveness Review No 177. (Prepared by the Minnesota Evidence-Based Practice Center under Contract No 290–2012–00016-I.) AHRQ Publication No 16-EHC019-EF. Rockville, MD, Agency for Healthcare Research and Quality, March 2016. Available at: www.effectivehealthcare.ahrq.gov/reports/final.cfm. Accessed May 2019.

Brodaty H: Realistic expectations for the management of Alzheimer's disease. Eur Neuropsychopharmacol 9(suppl 2):S43–S52, 1999 10332934

Brodaty H, Arasaratnam C: Meta-analysis of nonpharmacological interventions for neuropsychiatric symptoms of dementia. Am J Psychiatry 169(9):946–953, 2012 22952073

Chen Q, Ermann A, Shad MU: Effectiveness of dextromethorphan/quinidine in frontotemporal dementia. Am J Geriatr Psychiatry 26(4):506, 2018 29132987

Chien L-Y, Chu H, Guo J-L, et al: Caregiver support groups in patients with dementia: a meta-analysis. Int J Geriatr Psychiatry 26(10):1089–1098, 2011 21308785

Cipriani G, Lucetti C, Nuti A, et al: Wandering and dementia. Psychogeriatrics 14(2):135–142, 2014 24661471

Colling KB: Caregiver interventions for passive behaviors in dementia: links to the NDB model. Aging Ment Health 8(2):117–125, 2004 14982716

Connolly BS, Lang AE: Pharmacological treatment of Parkinson disease: a review. JAMA 311(16):1670–1683, 2014 24756517

Cooke JR, Ayalon L, Palmer BW, et al: Sustained use of CPAP slows deterioration of cognition, sleep, and mood in patients with Alzheimer's disease and obstructive sleep apnea: a preliminary study. J Clin Sleep Med 5(4):305–309, 2009 19968005

Cooper C, Tandy AR, Balamurali TBS, et al: A systematic review and meta-analysis of ethnic differences in use of dementia treatment, care, and research. Am J Geriatr Psychiatry 18(3):193–203, 2010 20224516

Cummings JL, Lyketsos CG, Peskind ER, et al: Effect of dextromethorphan-quinidine on agitation in patients with Alzheimer disease dementia: a randomized clinical trial. JAMA 314(12):1242–1254, 2015 26393847

Davies SJ, Burhan AM, Kim D, et al: Sequential drug treatment algorithm for agitation and aggression in Alzheimer's and mixed dementia. J Psychopharmacol 32(5):509–523, 2018 29338602

De Giorgi R, Series H: Treatment of inappropriate sexual behavior in dementia. Curr Treat Options Neurol 18(9):41, 2016 27511056

De Picker L, Van Den Eede F, Dumont G, et al: Antidepressants and the risk of hyponatremia: a class-by-class review of literature. Psychosomatics 55(6):536–547, 2014 25262043

Dolder CR, Davis LN, McKinsey J: Use of psychostimulants in patients with dementia. Ann Pharmacother 44(10):1624–1632, 2010 20736422

Droogsma E, van Asselt D, De Deyn PP: Weight loss and undernutrition in community-dwelling patients with Alzheimer's dementia: from population based studies to clinical management. Z Gerontol Geriatr 48(4):318–324, 2015 25990006

Farina N, Morrell L, Banerjee S: What is the therapeutic value of antidepressants in dementia? A narrative review. Int J Geriatr Psychiatry 32(1):32–49, 2017 27593707

Fleisher AS, Truran D, Mai JT, et al: Chronic divalproex sodium use and brain atrophy in Alzheimer disease. Neurology 77(13):1263–1271, 2011 21917762

Forbes D, Forbes SC, Blake CM, et al: Exercise programs for people with dementia. Cochrane Database Syst Rev (4):CD006489, 2015 25874613

Gilhooly KJ, Gilhooly MLM, Sullivan MP, et al: A meta-review of stress, coping and interventions in dementia and dementia caregiving. BMC Geriatr 16:106, 2016 27193287

Gitlin LN, Kales HC, Lyketsos CG: Nonpharmacologic management of behavioral symptoms in dementia. JAMA 308(19):2020–2029, 2012 23168825

Gitlin LN, Marx KA, Alonzi D, et al: Feasibility of the Tailored Activity Program for hospitalized (TAP-H) patients with behavioral symptoms. Gerontologist 57:575–584, 2016 27076056

Gitlin LN, Arthur P, Piersol C, et al: Targeting behavioral symptoms and functional decline in dementia: a randomized clinical trial. S Am Geriatr Soc 66(2):339–345, 2018 29192967

Gonyea JG, López LM, Velásquez EH: The effectiveness of culturally sensitive cognitive behavioral group intervention for Latino Alzheimer's caregivers. Gerontologist 56(2):292–302, 2016 24855313

Hansen BR, Hodgson NA, Budhathoki C, et al: Caregiver reactions to aggressive behaviors in persons with dementia in a diverse, community-dwelling sample. J Appl Gerontol 2018 29457520 [Epub ahead of print]

Hefti E, Blanco JG: Pharmacotherapeutic considerations for individuals with Down syndrome. Pharmacotherapy 37(2):214–220, 2017 27931082

Herrmann N, Black SE, Chow T, et al: Serotonergic function and treatment of behavioral and psychological symptoms of frontotemporal dementia. Am J Geriatr Psychiatry 20(9):789–797, 2012 21878805

Husebo BS, Ballard C, Cohen-Mansfield J, et al: The response of agitated behavior to pain management in persons with dementia. Am J Geriatr Psychiatry 22(7):708–717, 2014 23611363

Husebo BS, Achterberg W, Flo E: Identifying and managing pain in people with Alzheimer's disease and other types of dementia: a systematic review. CNS Drugs 30(6):481–497, 2016 27240869

Ito T, Meguro K, Akanuma K, et al: A randomized controlled trial of the group reminiscence approach in patients with vascular dementia. Dement Geriatr Cogn Disord 24(1):48–54, 2007 17565213

Jaïdi Y, Nonnonhou V, Kanagaratnam L, et al: Reduction of the anticholinergic burden makes it possible to decrease behavioral and psychological symptoms of dementia. Am J Geriatr Psychiatry 26(3):280–288, 2018 28890165

Jeste DV, Lacro JP, Bailey A, et al: Lower incidence of tardive dyskinesia with risperidone compared with haloperidol in older patients. J Am Geriatr Soc 47(6):716–719, 1999 10366172

Jeste DV, Blazer D, Casey D, et al: ACNP white paper: update on use of antipsychotic drugs in elderly persons with dementia. Neuropsychopharmacology 33(5):957–970, 2008 17637610

Jönsson AK, Schill J, Olsson H, et al: Venous thromboembolism during treatment with antipsychotics: a review of current evidence. CNS Drugs 32(1):47–64, 2018 29423659

Jorgensen LE, Messersmith JJ: Impact of aging and cognition on hearing assistive technology use. Semin Hear 36(3):162–174, 2015 27516716

Kales HC, Gitlin LN, Lyketsos CG, et al: Management of neuropsychiatric symptoms of dementia in clinical settings: recommendations from a multidisciplinary expert panel. J Am Geriatr Soc 62(4):762–769, 2014 24635665

Kales HC, Gitlin LN, Lyketsos CG: Assessment and management of behavioral and psychological symptoms of dementia. BMJ 350:h369, 2015 25731881

Kales HC, Gitlin LN, Stanislawski B, et al: Effect of the WeCareAdvisor™ on family caregiver outcomes in dementia: a pilot randomized controlled trial. BMC Geriatr 18(1):113, 2018 29747583

Kales HC, Lyketsos CG, Miller EM, Ballard C: Management of behavioral and psychological symptoms in people with Alzheimer's disease: an international Delphi consensus. Int Psychogeriatr 31(1):83–90, 2019 30068400

Kaster TS, Blumberger DM: Palliating severe refractory neuropsychiatric symptoms of dementia: is there a role for electroconvulsive therapy? Am J Geriatr Psychiatry 26(4):435–437, 2018 29428406

Katz IR, Rupnow M, Kozma C, et al: Risperidone and falls in ambulatory nursing home residents with dementia and psychosis or agitation: secondary analysis of a double-blind, placebo-controlled trial. Am J Geriatr Psychiatry 12(5):499–508, 2004 15353388

Kiosses DN, Alexopoulos GS: Problem-solving therapy in the elderly. Curr Treat Options Psychiatry 1(1):15–26, 2014 24729951

Kiosses DN, Rosenberg PB, McGovern A, et al: Depression and suicidal ideation during two psychosocial treatments in older adults with major depression and dementia. J Alzheimers Dis 48(2):453–462, 2015 26402009

Knol W, van Marum RJ, Jansen PA, et al: Antipsychotic drug use and risk of pneumonia in elderly people. J Am Geriatr Soc 56(4):661–666, 2008 18266664

Koch JM, Datta G, Makhdoom S, et al: Unmet visual needs of Alzheimer's disease patients in long-term care facilities. J Am Med Dir Assoc 6(4):233–237, 2005 16005408

Konovalov S, Muralee S, Tampi RR: Anticonvulsants for the treatment of behavioral and psychological symptoms of dementia: a literature review. Int Psychogeriatr 20(2):293–308, 2008 18047764

Kovach CR, Noonan PE, Schlidt AM, et al: A model of consequences of need-driven, dementia-compromised behavior. J Nurs Scholarsh 37(2):134–140, discussion 140, 2005 15960057

Lee EE, Chang B, Huege S, Hirst J: Complex clinical intersection: palliative care in patients with dementia. Am J Geriatr Psychiatry 26(2):224–234, 2018 28822692

Legere LE, McNeill S, Schindel Martin L, et al: Nonpharmacological approaches for behavioural and psychological symptoms of dementia in older adults: a systematic review of reviews. J Clin Nurs 27(7–8):e1360–e1376, 2018 28793380

Leontjevas R, Gerritsen DL, Smalbrugge M, et al: A structural multidisciplinary approach to depression management in nursing-home residents: a multicentre, stepped-wedge cluster-randomised trial. Lancet 381(9885):2255–2264, 2013 23643110

Leucht S, Cipriani A, Spineli L, et al: Comparative efficacy and tolerability of 15 antipsychotic drugs in schizophrenia: a multiple-treatments meta-analysis. Lancet 382(9896):951–962, 2013 23810019

Lichtwarck B, Tvera A-M, Roen I: Targeted Interdisciplinary Model for Evaluation and Treatment of Neuropsychiatric Symptoms—Manual, 2nd Edition. Ottestad, Norway, Centre for Old Age Psychiatric Research, Innlandet Hospital Trust, 2017

Lichtwarck B, Selbaek G, Kirkevold Ø, et al: Targeted interdisciplinary model for evaluation and treatment of neuropsychiatric symptoms: a cluster randomized controlled trial. Am J Geriatr Psychiatry 26(1):25–38, 2018 28669575

Liu J, Wang LN, Wu LY, et al: Treatment of epilepsy for people with Alzheimer's disease. Cochrane Database Syst Rev 11:CD011922, 2016 27805721

Livingston G, Kelly L, Lewis-Holmes E, et al: A systematic review of the clinical effectiveness and cost-effectiveness of sensory, psychological and behavioural interventions for managing agitation in older adults with dementia. Health Technol Assess 18(39):1–226, v–vi, 2014 24947468

Lonergan E, Luxenberg J: Valproate preparations for agitation in dementia. Cochrane Database Syst Rev (3):CD003945, 2009 19588348

Maglione M, Ruelaz Maher A, Hu J, et al: Off-Label Use of Atypical Antipsychotics: An Update. Comparative Effectiveness Review No 43. (Prepared by the Southern California Evidence-Based Practice Center under Contract No HHSA290-2007-10062-1.) AHRQ Publication No 11-EHC087-EF, Rockville, MD, Agency for Healthcare Research and Quality, September 2011

Maschi T, Kwak J, Ko E, et al: Forget me not: dementia in prison. Gerontologist 52(4):441–451, 2012 22230493

Maust DT, Kim HM, Seyfried LS, et al: Antipsychotics, other psychotropics, and the risk of death in patients with dementia: number needed to harm. JAMA Psychiatry 72(5):438–445, 2015 25786075

McCleery J, Cohen DA, Sharpley AL: Pharmacotherapies for sleep disturbances in dementia. Cochrane Database Syst Rev 11:CD009178, 2016 27851868

McCurry SM, Gibbons LE, Logsdon RG, et al: Nighttime insomnia treatment and education for Alzheimer's disease: a randomized, controlled trial. J Am Geriatr Soc 53(5):793–802, 2005 15877554

Minett TS, Thomas A, Wilkinson LM, et al: What happens when donepezil is suddenly withdrawn? An open label trial in dementia with Lewy bodies and Parkinson's disease with dementia. Int J Geriatr Psychiatry 18(11):988–993, 2003 14618549

Moran JA, Rafii MS, Keller SM, et al: The National Task Group on Intellectual Disabilities and Dementia Practices consensus recommendations for the evaluation and management of dementia in adults with intellectual disabilities. Mayo Clin Proc 88(8):831–840, 2013 23849993

Moretti R, Torre P, Antonello RM, et al: Olanzapine as a possible treatment of behavioral symptoms in vascular dementia: risks of cerebrovascular events: a controlled, open-label study. J Neurol 252(10):1186–1193, 2005 15809822

Nardell M, Tampi RR: Pharmacological treatments for frontotemporal dementias: a systematic review of randomized controlled trials. Am J Alzheimers Dis Other Demen 29(2):123–132, 2014 24164931

National Institute on Aging: Caring for a Person with Alzheimer's Disease: Your Easy-to-Use Guide. Bethesda, MD, National Institute on Aging, 2017. Available at: https://order.nia.nih.gov/publication/caring-for-a-person-with-alzheimers-disease-your-easy-to-use-guide. Accessed July 15, 2018.

Orgeta V, Qazi A, Spector A, et al: Psychological treatments for depression and anxiety in dementia and mild cognitive impairment: systematic review and meta-analysis. Br J Psychiatry 207(4):293–298, 2015 26429684

Oudman E: Is electroconvulsive therapy (ECT) effective and safe for treatment of depression in dementia? A short review. J ECT 28(1):34–38, 2012 22330702

Padala PR, Padala KP, Lensing SY, et al: Methylphenidate for apathy in community-dwelling older veterans with mild Alzheimer's disease: a double-blind, randomized, placebo-controlled trial. Am J Psychiatry 175(2):159–168, 2018 28945120

Palecek EJ, Teno JM, Casarett DJ, et al: Comfort feeding only: a proposal to bring clarity to decision-making regarding difficulty with eating for persons with advanced dementia. J Am Geriatr Soc 58(3):580–584, 2010 20398123

Peskind ER, Tsuang DW, Bonner LT, et al: Propranolol for disruptive behaviors in nursing home residents with probable or possible Alzheimer disease: a placebo-controlled study. Alzheimer Dis Assoc Disord 19(1):23–28, 2005 15764868

Porsteinsson AP, Antonsdottir IM: An update on the advancements in the treatment of agitation in Alzheimer's disease. Expert Opin Pharmacother 18(6):611–620, 2017 28300462

Rabins PV, Blacker D, Rovner BW, et al: American Psychiatric Association practice guideline for the treatment of patients with Alzheimer's disease and other dementias, second edition. Am J Psychiatry 164 (12 suppl):5–56, 2007

Reus VI, Fochtmann LJ, Eyler AE, et al: The American Psychiatric Association practice guideline on the use of antipsychotics to treat agitation or psychosis in patients with dementia. Am J Psychiatry 173(5):543–546, 2016 27133416

Rongen S, Kramers C, O'Mahony D, et al: Potentially inappropriate prescribing in older patients admitted to psychiatric hospital. Int J Geriatr Psychiatry 31(2):137–145, 2016 26032252

Rosenberg PB, Drye LT, Porsteinsson AP, et al: Change in agitation in Alzheimer's disease in the placebo arm of a nine-week controlled trial. Int Psychogeriatr 27(12):2059–2067, 2015 26305876

Ruthirakuhan MT, Herrmann N, Abraham EH, et al: Pharmacological interventions for apathy in Alzheimer's disease. Cochrane Database Syst Rev 5:CD012197, 2018 29727467

Satoh M, Ishikawa H, Meguro K, et al: Improved visual hallucination by donepezil and occipital glucose metabolism in dementia with Lewy bodies: the Osaki-Tajiri project. Eur Neurol 64(6):337–344, 2010 21071950

Scales K, Zimmerman S, Miller SJ: Evidence-based nonpharmacological practices to address behavioral and psychological symptoms of dementia. Gerontologist 58 (suppl 1):S88–S102, 2018 29361069

Schneider LS, Dagerman KS, Insel P: Risk of death with atypical antipsychotic drug treatment for dementia: meta-analysis of randomized placebo-controlled trials. JAMA 294(15):1934–1943, 2005 16234500

Schneider LS, Dagerman K, Insel PS: Efficacy and adverse effects of atypical antipsychotics for dementia: meta-analysis of randomized, placebo-controlled trials. Am J Geriatr Psychiatry 14(3):191–210, 2006a 16505124

Schneider LS, Tariot PN, Dagerman KS, et al: Effectiveness of atypical antipsychotic drugs in patients with Alzheimer's disease. N Engl J Med 355(15):1525–1538, 2006 17035647

Scoralick FM, Louzada LL, Quintas JL, et al: Mirtazapine does not improve sleep disorders in Alzheimer's disease: results from a double-blind, placebo-controlled pilot study. Psychogeriatrics 17(2):89–96, 2017 26818096

Segers K, Surquin M: Can mirtazapine counteract the weight loss associated with Alzheimer disease? A retrospective open-label study. Alzheimer Dis Assoc Disord 28(3):291–293, 2014 22760168

Seitz DP, Brisbin S, Herrmann N, et al: Efficacy and feasibility of nonpharmacological interventions for neuropsychiatric symptoms of dementia in long term care: a systematic review. J Am Med Dir Assoc 13(6):503–506.e2, 2012 22342481

Smith M, Gerdner LA, Hall GR, et al: History, development, and future of the progressively lowered stress threshold: a conceptual model for dementia care. J Am Geriatr Soc 52(10):1755–1760, 2004 15450057

Sparks MB: Inpatient care for persons with Alzheimer's disease. Crit Care Nurs Q 31(1):65–72, 2008 18316939

Stinton C, McKeith I, Taylor J-P, et al: Pharmacological management of Lewy body dementia: a systematic review and meta-analysis. Am J Psychiatry 172(8):731–742, 2015 26085043

Sultana J, Chang CK, Hayes RD, et al: Associations between risk of mortality and atypical antipsychotic use in vascular dementia: a clinical cohort study. Int J Geriatr Psychiatry 29(12):1249–1254, 2014 24633896

Sun F, Ong R, Burnette D: The influence of ethnicity and culture on dementia caregiving: a review of empirical studies on Chinese Americans. Am J Alzheimers Dis Other Demen 27(1):13–22, 2012 22467411

Surr CA, Griffiths AW, Kelley R: Implementing dementia care mapping as a practice development tool in dementia care services: a systematic review. Clin Interv Aging 13:165–177, 2018 29416325

Tampi RR, Tampi DJ: Efficacy and tolerability of benzodiazepines for the treatment of behavioral and psychological symptoms of dementia: a systematic review of randomized controlled trials. Am J Alzheimers Dis Other Demen 29(7):565–574, 2014 25551131

Tangwongchai S, Thavichachart N, Senanarong V, et al: Galantamine for the treatment of BPSD in Thai patients with possible Alzheimer's disease with or without cerebrovascular disease. Am J Alzheimers Dis Other Demen 23(6):593–601, 2008 18845693

Toot S, Devine M, Akporobaro A, Orrell M: Causes of hospital admission for people with dementia: a systematic review and meta-analysis. J Am Med Dir Assoc 14(7):463–470, 2013 23510826

U.S. Food and Drug Administration: FDA reinforces safety information about serious low blood sugar levels and mental health side effects with fluoroquinolone antibiotics; requires label changes. Food and Drug Administration Safety Announcement, July 10, 2018. Available at: https://www.fda.gov/Drugs/DrugSafety/ucm611032.htm. Accessed July 20, 2018.

van den Berg JF, Kruithof HC, Kok RM, et al: Electroconvulsive therapy for agitation and aggression in dementia: a systematic review. Am J Geriatr Psychiatry 26(4):419–434, 2018 29107460

Vandepitte S, Van Den Noortgate N, Putman K, et al: Effectiveness of supporting informal caregivers of people with dementia: a systematic review of randomized and non-randomized controlled trials. J Alzheimers Dis 52(3):929–965, 2016 27079704

van der Linde RM, Dening T, Stephan BCM, et al: Longitudinal course of behavioural and psychological symptoms of dementia: systematic review. Br J Psychiatry 209(5):366–377, 2016 27491532

Van Leeuwen E, Petrovic M, van Driel ML, et al: Withdrawal versus continuation of long-term antipsychotic drug use for behavioural and psychological symptoms in older people with dementia. Cochrane Database Syst Rev 3:CD007726, 2018 29605970

Vigen CL, Mack WJ, Keefe RS, et al: Cognitive effects of atypical antipsychotic medications in patients with Alzheimer's disease: outcomes from CATIE-AD. Am J Psychiatry 168(8):831–839, 2011 21572163

Viramontes TS, Truong H, Linnebur SA: Antidepressant-induced hyponatremia in older adults. Consult Pharm 31(3):139–150, 2016 26975593

Walaszek A: Ethical issues in the care of individuals with dementia, in Dementia. Edited by McNamara P. Santa Barbara, CA, ABC-CLIO, 2011, pp 123–150

Wang J, Yu J-T, Wang H-F, et al: Pharmacological treatment of neuropsychiatric symptoms in Alzheimer's disease: a systematic review and meta-analysis. J Neurol Neurosurg Psychiatry 86(1):101–109, 2015 24876182

Wang LY, Shofer JB, Rohde K, et al: Prazosin for the treatment of behavioral symptoms in patients with Alzheimer disease with agitation and aggression. Am J Geriatr Psychiatry 17(9):744–751, 2009 19700947

Williams K, Blyler D, Vidoni ED, et al: A randomized trial using telehealth technology to link caregivers with dementia care experts for in-home caregiving support: FamTechCare protocol. Res Nurs Health 41(3):219–227, 2018 29504666

Woerner MG, Correll CU, Alvir JM, et al: Incidence of tardive dyskinesia with risperidone or olanzapine in the elderly: results from a 2-year, prospective study in antipsychotic-naïve patients. Neuropsychopharmacology 36(8):1738–1746, 2011 21508932

Young JJ, Lavakumar M, Tampi D, et al: Frontotemporal dementia: latest evidence and clinical implications. Ther Adv Psychopharmacol 8(1):33–48, 2018 29344342

Zubenko GS, Sommers BR, Cohen BM: On the marketing and use of pharmacogenetic tests for psychiatric treatment. JAMA Psychiatry 75(8):769–770, 2018 29799933

CHAPTER 6

MANAGEMENT OF OTHER THREATS TO SAFETY

Précis

Because of the cognitive and functional impairments of persons with dementia, they and their family members may encounter many threats to their safety. In Chapter 5, I discussed managing the risks associated with physical aggression and wandering. In this chapter, I cover a wide range of other safety concerns, including falls (probably the greatest threat to the independence of an older adult), fires, driving, financial exploitation, medication nonadherence (including refusing medications), refusing assistance with activities of daily living (ADLs), hoarding, and the risk of injury related to access to firearms and other household dangers. As always, educating and supporting caregivers are critical to help them address these threats to safety.

FALLS

As noted in the section "Assessing and Supporting Activities of Daily Living" in Chapter 2, persons with dementia face a high risk of falls. About one-third of community-dwelling older adults fall each year, and for persons with dementia, the rate is as high as 50%–80% per year (Burton et al. 2015). In addition to cognitive impairment, risk factors for falling include gait, strength, or balance deficits; sensory deficits; acute illnesses; medications; footwear; assistive devices; alcohol; factors within the home; and caregiver factors (Phelan et al. 2015). Falls account for a large percentage of the injuries that persons with dementia sustain; falls can lead to bone fractures, hospitalization, and institutionalization (Rowe and Fehrenbach 2004). The U.S. Centers for Disease Control and Prevention (CDC), adopting the

American Geriatrics Society and the British Geriatrics Society guidelines for preventing falls, have made available a toolkit for patients, caregivers, and clinicians to screen for and address the risk of falling (Centers for Disease Control and Prevention 2017; see also the section "Resources for Patients, Families, and Caregivers" at the end of this chapter).

The CDC recommends that clinicians review a patient's medications and stop or reduce to the lowest effective dosage those medications that could increase the risk of falling. These include anticonvulsants, antidepressants, antipsychotics, benzodiazepines, opioids, sedative-hypnotics, anticholinergics, antihistamines, antihypertensives, and muscle relaxants. Physical assessment should include checking for orthostatic hypotension (systolic blood pressure drop >20 mmHg or diastolic blood pressure drop >10 mmHg within 3 minutes of standing), a visual acuity test, cardiac examination, neurological examination, musculoskeletal examination (including feet), and gait assessment using the Timed Up and Go (TUG) test or something similar (Phelan et al. 2015). (The TUG test involves asking the patient to stand up from a chair, walk 10 feet, then return to the chair; an older adult who takes 12 seconds or longer to do so is at risk of falling.)

The clinician should consider referral to a physical therapist to improve a patient's gait, strength, and balance; to develop a home exercise program for the patient; and to recommend, select, and fit an assistive device if indicated (Phelan et al. 2015). Home-based exercise and group exercise programs, taking place one to five times per week for 3–12 months, appear to be effective for persons with dementia, reducing their risk of falling by 32% (Burton et al. 2015). The elements of a successful exercise program include strength, balance, and endurance work; progression of intensity over time; engaging caregivers; tailoring exercises to participants' preferences; and offering a choice of exercises (Burton et al. 2015). Parenthetically, exercise may also be the most effective intervention for delaying functional decline in persons with dementia—another reason to recommend exercise (Laver et al. 2016).

The clinician should consider vitamin D supplementation, cholecalciferol 1,000 IU/day (Phelan et al. 2015). Orthostatic hypotension can be addressed by lowering dosages of antihypertensive medications, stopping medications that can cause orthostasis, recommending above-the-knee support hose, and having the patient sleep with the head of the bed elevated (Phelan et al. 2015).

It is critical to engage caregivers who can modify the home environment to make walking in the home safer, who can help the person with dementia complete recommended exercises, and who can ensure that the person with demen-

TABLE 6–1.	Advice for family caregivers to address the risk of falling

Talk with your loved one and his or her health care provider about preventing falls.

Tell a health care provider right away if your loved one has fallen, seems unsteady, or is worried about falling.

Keep an up-to-date list of your loved one's medication. Reviewing the medication list is an important part of reducing the risk of falling.

Ask the health care provider about vitamin D to increase bone health.

Encourage your loved one to keep moving.

Activities that improve balance and strengthen the legs help reduce the risk of falling.

Staying active also helps your loved one feel more confident about walking.

Check with the health care provider about what type of exercise is best for your loved one.

Have your loved one's eyes and feet checked.

Your loved one should have eyesight checked at least once a year.

Replace eyeglasses as needed.

Ask the health care provider to check your loved one's feet at least once a year.

Discuss proper footwear, and ask whether your loved one should be referred to a foot specialist.

Make the home a safer place for walking.

Keep the floors free of clutter.

Remove throw rugs or use double-sided tape to keep rugs from slipping.

Add grab bars in the bathroom: one in the tub and one next to the toilet.

Install handrails and lights on all staircases.

Make sure the home has lots of light.

Source. Adapted from Centers for Disease Control and Prevention 2017.

tia is consistently using an assistive device (Phelan et al. 2015). Table 6–1 summarizes the CDC's recommendations for family caregivers to help prevent falls.

Home safety assessment and modification and gradual reduction of psychotropic medications were found to be effective in community-dwelling older adults without dementia (Gillespie et al. 2012), but it is not clear whether these findings would apply to persons with dementia. An in-home occupational therapy assessment may identify safety concerns inside the home (clutter or obstacles, loose rugs or slippery surfaces, lack of handrails on stairs, poor lighting, ill-fitting shoes, unsuitable assistive devices) or outside the home (cracked pavement, sloped yards); such an assessment may also identify concerns related to how the person with dementia performs mobility-related tasks (Phelan et al. 2015).

A wearable medical alert device may allow a person who has fallen to seek assistance, but the cognitive impairment of a person with dementia limits applicability; a wearable automated fall detector does not require activation by the person with dementia who has fallen, but there are very few studies of such devices in real-world settings and none in persons with dementia (Chaudhuri et al. 2014). Wearable activity monitors (e.g., Fitbit) and smartphone-based or smartwatch-based apps may eventually be helpful, but they have not been vetted in persons with dementia.

COOKING AND FIRE SAFETY

The following safety issues can arise when caring for a person with dementia:

- Memory loss and executive dysfunction can result in problems with preparing meals, including leaving the stove on too long, putting inappropriate objects into a microwave, and burning food.
- If someone in the household, including the person with dementia, smokes, then smoking products and matches can pose a hazard.
- In the event of a fire, a person with dementia may not be able to get help.

Cooking is the leading cause of home fires and home injuries, and older adults are at higher risk of dying from a cooking-related fires: 28% of all people fatally injured in fires are older adults (Electrical Safety Foundation International 2015). As detailed in Table 6–2, there are a number of steps that family members should take to reduce the risk of a fire.

One way to increase fire safety is for persons with dementia and other members of the household to quit smoking. Persons with dementia are less likely to be prescribed nicotine replacement than those without dementia: more than 97.5% of smokers with dementia have not been prescribed nicotine replacement, varenicline, or bupropion (Huang et al. 2013). However, tobacco cessation should be encouraged in order to increase quality of life, decrease respiratory symptoms (which could cause distress), improve cardiac function, reduce disability, and reduce the risk of fire (Cataldo and Glantz 2010).

In the updated Dementia Management Quality Measurement Set, the American Academy of Neurology (AAN) and the American Psychiatric

---

TABLE 6–2. Advice for family caregivers to reduce the risk of a fire

Display emergency numbers and the home address next to all telephones.

Install functioning smoke alarms and carbon monoxide detectors in the kitchen and all sleeping areas. Use alarms with a flashing light if the person with dementia or other family members have hearing loss. Check batteries regularly.

Do not keep flammable and volatile materials near gas appliances or a gas pilot.

Install child safety knobs and automatic shutoff switch on stove, or remove the knobs for the stove.

Consider disconnecting the stove or installing a hidden gas valve or circuit breaker on the stove so that the person with dementia cannot turn it on.

If a grill is accessible, remove the fuel source and fire starter.

Do not leave the person with dementia home alone with a fire in the fireplace.

Do not use electric mattress pads, blankets, and sheets.

Make sure there is a functioning fire extinguisher in the home.

Matches, lighters, ashtrays, cigarettes, and other means of smoking should be removed from view. If the person with dementia does smoke, make sure the person is supervised.

Routinely check cords, outlets, switches, and appliances for signs of damage. Do not use damaged electrical devices. Do not use extension cords permanently and never with major appliances. Do not overload electrical outlets.

If the person with dementia or other family members use walkers or wheelchairs, make sure that they will fit through doorways.

Have a fire escape plan. Assign a family member or other caregiver to assist the person with dementia in safely getting out of the house in the event of an emergency.

Source. These recommendations are based on a review and summary of the information provided by the following: Alzheimer's Association (2018a), Electrical Safety Foundation International (2015), and National Institute on Aging (2017b).

Association (APA) recommend annual screening for environmental risks to the patient and, for patients screening positive, steps to mitigate such risks (Sanders et al. 2017). I believe these risks include falls (discussed in the previous section), fire safety, and the other hazards covered in the section on firearms later in this chapter.

DRIVING SAFETY

Persons with dementia and even mild cognitive impairment (MCI) are at much higher risk of getting into a motor vehicle accident than older adults without (Rabins et al. 2007). Half of patients with MCI (CDR [Clinical Dementia Rating instrument] score of 0.5) stop driving within 6 years, and half of patients with mild dementia (CDR score of 1) are no longer driving within 2 years (Stout et al. 2018). Neither patients, families, nor clinicians may be reliable judges of the ability of a patient with cognitive impairment to drive safely (Bixby et al. 2015). No simple bedside screening test has been found to reliably detect unsafe driving; even composite batteries lack necessary sensitivity and specificity, and their complexity may prevent clinicians from adopting them (Bennett et al. 2016). Predictors of driving risk include history of a crash in the past 1–5 years, history of a traffic citation in the past 2–3 years, caregiver report of safety concerns, reduced mileage (<60 miles per week) due to self-imposed or externally imposed restrictions (e.g., not driving at night, not driving in the rain), and aggressive or impulsive personality (Iverson et al. 2010). Clinicians should also ask whether the person has gotten lost while driving. Other factors to consider include vision, hearing, head-turning ability, daytime sleepiness, parkinsonism, neuropathy, symptomatic cardiac disease, seizures, poorly controlled diabetes, and alcohol use (Carter et al. 2015; Rabins et al. 2007). Distracted driving may have more of an impact on older adults than younger adults.

Patients and family members should be informed about the risks associated with driving with MCI and dementia (Rabins et al. 2007). The AAN and APA's Dementia Management Quality Measurement Set recommends annual screening for driving risks and, for patients screening positive, informing about alternatives to driving (Sanders et al. 2017). See Table 6–3 for a description of CDR scoring, which is relevant to stratifying risk.

Patients with MCI (CDR of 0.5) and mild dementia (CDR of 1) should be encouraged to voluntarily stop driving or otherwise undergo a professional driving evaluation conducted by an occupational therapist who is a certified driver rehabilitation specialist or at a local agency; the strength of the recommendation should be proportional to the number of risk factors, as described above. Family members should be encouraged to ensure that a patient with dementia is still able to get around even after he or she is no longer allowed to drive (Iverson et al. 2010). Patients with moderate and severe dementia (CDR of 2 and 3, respectively) should not be allowed to drive (Rabins et al. 2007). Laws regarding the reporting of concerns about driving vary among jurisdictions around the world (Carter et al. 2015); clinicians should become familiar with their local laws. It may be necessary for family members, as a last resort, to take away car keys, disable the car, or remove the car (Rabins et al. 2007). Even if a patient is deemed safe to drive now, reassessment should take place every 6 months (Iverson et al. 2010).

TABLE 6–3. CDR (Clinical Dementia Rating instrument) for use in addressing safety issues

Score	Cognition	Functioning
0.5	Mild problems with memory or other cognitive domains, with objective deficits on testing; no problem with orientation	No significant functional decline, but completing instrumental ADLs may require more effort; perhaps slight impairment with respect to community affairs and hobbies
1	Moderate memory loss (especially recent events); mild problems with orientation; mild problems with executive function, but social functioning intact	Problems with finances, preparing a complex meal, or maintaining a difficult medication schedule; may need prompting for personal ADLs
2	Severe memory loss, with new material rapidly lost; usually disoriented to time, often to place; severe problems with executive function; social functioning impaired	Problems with household tasks and preparing a simple meal; requires assistance with personal ADLs; still can go to functions outside of home but not independently
3	Severe memory loss; oriented only to person; unable to make judgments or solve problems	Requires considerable assistance with personal ADLs; cannot go to functions outside of home

Note. See text discussions for application of the CDR to assessing the risk associated with driving and with having access to a firearm in the home.
ADLs = activities of daily living.
Source. Morris 1993; Rabins et al. 2007.

Recommending that someone stop driving can be a very difficult conversation for patients, family members, and clinicians. Losing the ability to drive can have significant psychological impact (e.g., as a marker of loss of independence) and psychosocial implications (e.g., decreased access to supports). Discussions should be nonjudgmental, should focus on facts, and could appeal to the person's sense of conscientiousness (i.e., not wanting to injure someone else). Family members will need to be encouraged and supported throughout the process. They may find the Health in Aging and National Highway Traffic Safety Administration (NHTSA) websites listed in the "Resources for Patients, Families, and Caregivers" section at the end of this chapter to be helpful. Clinicians can find a more comprehensive discussion of the topic of driving safety for older adults in the *Clinician's Guide to*

Assessing and Counseling Older Drivers, available on the American Geriatrics Society and NHTSA websites (Pomidor 2016). Case Example 6–1 presents a case of a person at heightened risk of motor vehicle accident due to dementia.

Case Example 6–1: "If She Can't Drive, Who's Going to Take Her Shopping?"

Mrs. Muller is a 74-year-old widow, living alone in the same house she has occupied for the past 30 years. Last year, she was diagnosed with major neurocognitive disorder due to Alzheimer's disease after presenting with a 2-year history of memory loss and word-finding difficulties. She was thought to be in an early stage of dementia, and she appeared to be able to take care of herself, with some assistance from her adult son who lives in the area. Specifically, he set up weekly pill boxes for her and, with her permission, changed her bills to automatic payment. She presents for a routine annual medical appointment to her primary care physician. Neither she nor her son has any concerns about how she is doing.

Aware of the risk of driving for persons with even mild dementia, the physician asks Mrs. Muller and her son if they are worried about her driving. They are not, although her son would prefer that Mrs. Muller no longer drive his children to the ice cream shop. Her son drove her to the appointment today. They note that about 1 year ago, she scraped the side of the car when parking the car in her garage. Three months ago, she accidentally drove over a barrier in a parking lot, resulting in extensive repairs. Mrs. Muller drives about three times per week: to purchase groceries, to get her hair done, and to socialize with friends at lunch. She no longer drives at night because she got disoriented once and had a hard time getting home. She carries a cell phone with her and thinks that she could call her son for help if she needed to, and he concurs. She has not had any traffic violations. Both she and her son feel that she can drive safely as long as she stays on familiar routes during the daytime.

The physician reviews the risk of motor vehicle accidents for persons with dementia and recommends that Mrs. Muller stop driving. Both Mrs. Muller and her son raise objections, stating that the two accidents have been minor and have resulted in no injuries and that she has had the good judgment of limiting her driving. They are worried that she will become isolated and lonely if she is not allowed to drive. Her son is very busy with work and his own children and would not be able to drive her regularly. They insist that she will be able to drive safely and promise to call the physician if they have any concerns.

The physician validates Mrs. Muller's fears about losing her driving privileges and her feeling that she is slowly losing her independence and her mind. The physician acknowledges the stress her son feels as a caregiver with multiple other responsibilities and appeals to their sense of conscientiousness and not wanting to be harmed or harm others in an accident. Recognizing that bedside assessment is not accurate, the physician recommends that she be evaluated by an occupational therapist who is also a certified driver rehabilitation specialist. If the occupational therapist identifies any safety concerns, Mrs. Muller will need to cease driving; if not, the issue needs to be revisited in 6 months because her driving ability will change over time. In the meantime, the physician asks Mrs. Muller and her son to begin exploring alternatives to her driving, such as a local transportation service for seniors. Mrs. Muller has not had her eyes examined in several years, and so a referral is made for an eye examination as a way of addressing any correctable impediments to driving. Mrs. Muller hesitantly agrees to this plan and agrees to follow up in 1 month after the occupational therapist's evaluation has taken place.

FINANCIAL INCAPACITY AND RISK OF EXPLOITATION

Problems with managing one's finances are common even in mild dementia (prevalence of incapacity is 47%–87%) and are nearly universal in moderate dementia (90%–100%) (Marson et al. 2000). Detecting financial incapacity can be challenging, because patients and their families often underestimate or do not recognize impairment (Marson 2013). As discussed in the section "Assessing and Supporting Activities of Daily Living" in Chapter 2, clinicians should educate patients and their family members about financial incapacity and recommend that appropriate planning takes place (e.g., setting up a durable financial power of attorney).

Elder financial fraud and scams are common, affecting 5.6%–6% of older adults (Burnes et al. 2017). Risk factors for financial exploitation of older adults in the United States include being African American, poverty, increasing number of nonspousal household members, and having at least one impairment in instrumental ADLs; living with a spouse or partner is protective (Peterson et al. 2014). Clinicians should warn family members about the possibility of financial exploitation and ask them to watch carefully for any evidence of this (Rabins et al. 2007). Of course, family members themselves can exploit persons with dementia, a situation that may be particularly difficult for clinicians to identify and address (Marson 2013).

Clinicians should maintain a high index of suspicion for financial incapacity; they should ask patients and family members about warning signs such as forgetting to pay bills or paying the same one twice, misplacing financial documents, becoming confused about financial terms, developing problems with math, and becoming interested in financial solicitations that could be scams (Marson 2013). In complex situations, such as when there is family conflict over finances, formal assessment of financial capacity by a neuropsychologist, geriatric psychologist, or forensic psychiatrist may be necessary (Marson 2013).

Financial exploitation of older adults is a form of elder abuse, which is discussed in the section "Protecting the Vulnerable Elder With Dementia" in Chapter 7. Depending on the laws of the local jurisdiction, clinicians may need to report suspected financial exploitation to appropriate authorities (Rabins et al. 2007).

ADHERENCE TO MEDICATIONS

Managing a complex medication regimen to address multiple medical issues can be challenging for anyone, let alone a person with dementia. Safety issues can arise when a person with dementia forgets to take medications, takes medications at the wrong times, takes the wrong medications, takes excessive doses of medications, or refuses to take medications. Visual impairment, neuropathy, and problems with manual dexterity may interfere with adherence (Elliott et al. 2015). Persons with dementia may refuse medications because of their taste, because of side effects, because of paranoid ideation (e.g., fear that they are being poisoned), or because doing so may hasten the end of life (Elliott et al. 2015; Haskins and Wick 2017). As dementia advances, patients may have difficulty swallowing medications. Problems with adherence can lead to medical harm, including hospitalization (Elliott et al. 2015). All of these adherence issues can have a significant effect on caregivers as well (Aston et al. 2017).

Clinicians should ensure that family caregivers have adequate knowledge about the risks and benefits of medications because this may help caregivers encourage the person with dementia to adhere to their medication regimen; clinicians should employ a collaborative approach involving the patient and family caregivers (Aston et al. 2017). Pill boxes (set up by the patient under supervision, by a family member, or by a pharmacy), blister packaging, and automated pill dispensers may improve adherence but tend to become less effective as dementia becomes more severe; patients may also resist adopting these approaches (Aston et al. 2017). Advice for family caregivers regarding promoting medication adherence and other medication safety issues is listed in Table 6–4.

One response to medication refusal in long-term care is to covertly administer medications to persons with dementia, typically by crushing or dissolving the medication or by hiding it in food. It is estimated that this practice takes place in 43%–71% of nursing homes and that 1.5%–17% of

TABLE 6–4. Advice for family caregivers to promote medication safety

Know what medications your loved one is taking.

Keep a list of all medications, including over-the-counter medications, vitamins, and supplements. For each medication, list the reason for taking it, the prescriber, the dosage, its color and shape, and time(s) the medication is taken.

Keep a list of allergies.

Bring the medication list and allergy list to all medical appointments. Update the medication list when changes are made.

Ask the primary care provider or pharmacist to regularly review the list to make sure that all the medications are still needed and to check for any interactions. Ask if any medications can be safely discontinued.

For each medication, ask why it is being used, what positive effects to expect, what side effects to watch for, how long it will need to be taken, what the dosage is, what time(s) of day it should be taken, and what to do if a dose is missed.

Some medications may require periodic blood tests. Make sure the primary care provider explains this to you.

Help make sure that your loved one is taking medications correctly.

Keep the list of medications handy. Maintain a daily routine for taking medications and try to do so in a calm environment.

As dementia progresses, your loved one will need more help remembering to take medications. Use simple and clear instructions.

Use a weekly pill box to keep track of medications. At first, your loved one could fill it, under your supervision, or you could fill it together. Later, you may need to take over filling the pill box.

Consider asking the pharmacy to use blister packs to make it easier to track adherence to medications. (There may be a fee.) Consider using an automated pill dispenser or a pill box with alarms.

If a dose is missed accidentally, call your loved one's primary care provider and ask what to do.

If troubling side effects occur, contact the primary care provider.

You may need to lock up medications so that your loved one does not take extra doses accidentally. Dispose of medications that are no longer used or that are expired.

Keep the number for poison control center handy. If you think that your loved one has overdosed on medication, call 911 or poison control center.

TABLE 6–4.   Advice for family caregivers to promote medication
safety *(continued)*

Know what to do if your loved one is refusing medications.

Don't force the issue. Stop, and try again 10–15 minutes later. Be reassuring and calm and explain what you are doing.

Contact your loved one's primary care provider and ask what to do.

If you think that your loved one would do better taking medications at a different time of day, or less frequently, discuss this with the primary care provider.

Try to figure out what might be causing the medication refusal: Is your loved one experiencing side effects? Does the pill taste bad? Is your loved one having trouble swallowing? Is your loved one suspicious about the pills (maybe afraid of being poisoned)? Has your loved one given up on life and decided to quit taking medications?

If swallowing is a problem, ask the primary care provider if one or more of the medications are available as a dissolvable tablet, liquid, or patch.

Do not crush or dissolve or hide medications in food without talking with your primary care provider.

Source.   These recommendations are based on a review and summary of the information provided by the following: Allen (2017), Alzheimer's Association (2018b), and National Institute on Aging (2017b).

nursing home residents have received medications covertly (Young and Unger 2016). Covert administration of medications raises ethical concerns, might constitute elder abuse, and may have legal implications (Hung et al. 2012). The core ethical issue is whether administering a medication covertly in the best interest of the patient outweighs the harms of deceiving the patient, the risks of the patient not receiving the intervention, and the benefits of an alternate intervention (Hung et al. 2012; Young and Unger 2016). The U.K. Royal College of Psychiatrists' statement on this topic argues that covert administration is acceptable in certain circumstances—namely, when there is clear benefit from covert administration, when there are significant harms from not doing so, and when the patient is unable to understand the situation and is unable to learn (i.e., does not have medical decision-making capacity) (Royal College of Psychiatrists 2004). Clinicians considering covert administration of medications may take the steps described in Table 6–5 to help determine if this approach is appropriate. Clinicians should of course be aware of and follow local laws and regulations before recommending this approach.

TABLE 6–5.	Steps for clinicians to take when considering covert medication administration

1. Determine that the patient does not have the capacity to participate in this medical decision. If the patient has decisional capacity, covert administration of medication is not appropriate.

2. Carefully weigh the benefits of the medication being administered covertly against the risks of the patient not receiving the medication. If there are reasonable alternatives to covert administration, try those first.

3. Determine that covert administration is likely to be safer and more effective than alternate approaches.

4. Determine whether crushing and/or dissolving the medication will affect its efficacy, perhaps in consultation with a pharmacist.

5. Consider seeking ethical or legal consultation.

6. Explain risks, benefits, and alternatives of covert medication administration to the patient's proxy decision maker, and obtain consent from that person.

7. Work collaboratively with the staff of the long-term care facility on implementing the plan to covertly administer a medication.

8. Document this process in the medical record.

9. Regularly review whether covert medication administration is still necessary.

Note. Clinicians should always follow pertinent laws and regulations and seek consultation as needed.
Source. Royal College of Psychiatrists 2004; Young and Unger 2016.

REFUSAL OF ASSISTANCE WITH ACTIVITIES OF DAILY LIVING

A key goal of dementia care is keeping persons with dementia in their own homes as long as possible, which entails offering more support for ADLs. Some persons with dementia resist the notion that they need help with their ADLs and may ultimately refuse to accept help, which in turn can threaten their ability to stay in their own homes. The prevalence of care refusal among community-dwelling persons with dementia may be as high as 27% (Ishii et al. 2010). Refusal of care can also be a significant issue in long-term care facilities (prevalence of 9%–19%), where unfamiliar staff care for persons with moderate and severe dementia. Bathing, toileting, grooming, dressing, and attempts to redirect the person with dementia can trigger refusal of care (Ishii et al. 2010). Persons with dementia may refuse care verbally, may get into arguments, may resist physically, or may become combative, thereby frustrating and potentially endangering formal caregivers and family members (Ishii et al. 2010). As with other behavioral and psychological symptoms of dementia, refusal of care fluctuates substantially over time (Konno et al. 2014).

The clinician assessing a patient who has been refusing care should consider the possibility of pain, depression, delusions, or delirium (Ishii et al. 2010) and address these as discussed in Chapter 5. Playing prerecorded music during ADLs may reduce refusal of care; the music should either be relaxing or based on the patient's preferences (Konno et al. 2014). Training formal caregivers in a person-centered approach to bathing (namely, respecting privacy and increasing comfort) may reduce refusal of assistance with bathing (Konno et al. 2014). Case Example 6–2 describes the approach to a patient who is refusing care at home.

Case Example 6–2: "There's No Way They're Going to Let Someone in."

Mr. Jeong is an 88-year-old married man with mixed dementia (with elements of Alzheimer's disease and vascular dementia), which has been progressing slowly over the past 5 years. He and his wife—under pressure from their children, who were concerned about their ability to care for themselves—moved into a "senior living apartment" 3 years ago. Mrs. Jeong is cognitively intact but has significant problems related to arthritis and congestive heart failure; she is responsible for all household chores but has been less able to do these because of pain and fatigue. Mr. Jeong is either unable or unwilling to help. According to his children, he has become "bitter and resentful" since moving into the apartment, and he has refused to allow any paid caregivers or housekeepers into the apartment. Mr. Jeong children call the primary care provider to vent their frustration with his not accepting in-home services. The primary care provider reviews Mr. Jeong chart and collects collateral information from the family.

Formerly an avid reader and follower of current events, Mr. Jeong now has very limited interests, simply watching game shows on television all day, leading his children to wonder if he is depressed. Mrs. Jeong has reported that he sometimes refuses to take his medications, leading to repeated arguments between husband and wife, but no physical altercations; he has expressed feeling "overmedicated" and wants to take fewer medications. He also gets upset when his wife prompts him to bathe more frequently or chides him on his choice of clothing. Mr. Jeong stopped driving years ago and never managed the finances or prepared meals. There are no firearms in the home. He enjoys drinking whiskey, and his wife and children wonder if perhaps he is drinking too much because he is unsteady on his feet after a drink or two.

In addition to mixed dementia, Mr. Jeong has dyslipidemia, which is well controlled with atorvastatin. He has a history of hypertension and is taking hydrochlorothiazide and atenolol, with systolic blood pressures consistently in the 100–110 range and heart rate in the 50–60 range, but no orthostatic hypotension. He also takes donepezil 10 mg/day, several vitamins each day, and occasional acetaminophen for neck pain; he may also be taking a traditional Korean remedy, though this is unclear. He has denied suicidal ideation and paranoia but has endorsed low energy and lack of motivation. His wife feels he is sleeping too much. Mrs. Jeong denies feeling depressed herself but admits to feeling very frustrated. Their children are worried about her physical health and concerned that she may not be adequately caring for herself. There is no evidence of physical abuse, neglect, or financial exploitation.

Mr. Jeoong primary care provider identifies the following areas of concern for this patient with major neurocognitive disorder of moderate severity: 1) depression and/or apathy, 2) caregiver burnout, 3) polypharmacy, 4) medication nonadherence, 5) excessive alcohol use, 6) increased risk of falls, and 7) need for increased support in the home. There appear to be no concerns with elder abuse, fire safety, driving safety, or access to firearms. Whether Mr. Jeong has the capacity to make medical decisions is unclear, but this is not an immediately pressing issue.

Given the complexity of the situation, the primary care provider schedules a 45-minute appointment and invites Mrs. Jeong and the couple's children to attend or participate by phone. The clinic social worker will participate in the appointment and will be available for additional consultation afterward. The goals of this conference with Mr. Jeong and his family will be to highlight and address the concerns identified and to ensure that Mr. and Mrs. Jeong have adequate support at home.

Refusing to eat and drink may represent the final stage of dementia. This refusal can be challenging for family members to witness, who may need education and support regarding end-of-life care for persons with dementia. Insertion of feeding tubes and intravenous administration of fluids cause discomfort without apparent benefit and should not be done.

HOARDING

Although by DSM-5 definition (American Psychiatric Association 2013), persons with dementia do not meet criteria for *hoarding disorder*, *hoarding behaviors* are common among persons with dementia, with 25% of community-dwelling day care participants, 23% of geriatric psychiatric inpatients, and 15% of nursing home residents affected (Ayers et al. 2015). A person with hoarding disorder earlier in life could go on to develop dementia, which may exacerbate the symptoms of hoarding disorder. Dementia-related hoarding behaviors such as collecting, stealing, or hiding objects are usually related to cognitive impairments and disinhibition and may be associated with agitation (Ayers et al. 2015). Persons with the behavioral variant of frontotemporal dementia may be at higher risk of hoarding (Frank and Misiaszek 2012). Hoarding can lead to social isolation, an increased risk of falling, problems with medication adherence, problems with food safety (spoiled or contaminated food), poor hygiene and other functional impairments, infestation with insects or rodents, fire hazards, exacerbation of medical problems, and even eviction from home (Ayers et al. 2015). The insight of persons with dementia tends to be poor, leading to challenges in treatment.

Treatment includes addressing any comorbidities that could be contributing to hoarding behavior, including depression, psychosis, obsessions, and compulsions. Preliminary evidence suggests that psychotherapeutic approaches, including cognitive-behavioral therapy, motivational interviewing, cognitive rehabilitation, and exposure therapy, may be helpful (Ayers et al. 2015). Treatment may need to be more intense than typical psychotherapy: one protocol involved an average of 35 weekly in-home sessions (Ayers et al. 2015). There are almost no studies of psychopharmacological interventions for hoarding disorder in persons with dementia. I would recommend an empirical approach—namely, considering a selective serotonin reuptake inhibitor if depression, obsessions, compulsions, or impulsivity are present and an antipsychotic if psychosis is present.

Some communities may have agencies or organizations that can help individuals with hoarding disorder "dig out" of their homes; people with dementia may not have the capacity, however, to appreciate the risks of their situation and agree to receiving help (Frank and Misiaszek 2012). In extreme cases, hoarding may constitute elder abuse (specifically, self-neglect), which may require intervention from a social services agency.

FIREARMS, POWER TOOLS, AND OTHER HOUSEHOLD DANGERS

In the United States, 39% of people age 55 years and older report having at least one firearm in the home (with significant regional variation), and about one-fifth of firearm owners report having left the firearm loaded and unlocked sometime in the past year (Lum et al. 2016). A diagnosis of dementia in and of itself does not mean that the person with dementia cannot safely live in a home with a firearm. However, as dementia progresses, the risk of harm to the person with dementia and others in the home grows. For example, 91% of all elder suicides are by firearm (Betz et al. 2018). Disinhibition, confusion, and paranoia could affect patients' behavior with respect to firearms, potentially putting themselves, their family members, and other people who enter the home at risk (Betz et al. 2018).

Clinicians should screen all persons with dementia for the presence of a firearm in the home (Betz et al. 2018). The clinician should ask about depression, suicidal ideation, homicidal ideation, and paranoia; the presence of any of these should lead the clinician to recommend removing the firearm from the home, at least until the symptoms have resolved. Persons with moderate or severe dementia (CDR score 2 or 3, respectively) should not have access to a firearm (Betz et al. 2018). When a person is diagnosed with MCI (CDR 0.5) or mild dementia (CDR 1), the clinician should discuss the risk of accidental or intentional injury or death with the person and family members. The patient and family should be counseled regarding restricting access, for example, via a trigger lock, keeping the firearm locked up, keeping ammunition locked up separately from the firearm, or removing the firearm from the home (Betz et al. 2018). Persons with dementia and their family should consider a "firearm retirement date" (Betz et al. 2018). Like discussions about driving safety, these discussions can be emotional and challenging. The clinician may need to notify local authorities if the patient refuses to allow a restriction and if there is a risk of harm (Betz et al. 2018).

There may be other dangers in the home. Family members should be advised to lock up power tools and other machinery; remove poisonous plants from the home; keep fish tanks out of reach; restrict access to a swimming pool; keep electrical cords out of the way and cover electrical outlets with childproof plugs; lock up alcohol; lock up household cleaning products, knives, scissors, and small appliances; lower hot water temperature; and place red tape around vents, radiators, and heating devices to hopefully serve as a deterrent for touching them (Alzheimer's Association 2018a). I have had patients injure themselves accidentally by trying to climb a ladder or step stool, so I would suggest removing ladders and step stools from the home or locking them away.

SUMMARY: ENSURING THE SAFETY OF A PERSON WITH DEMENTIA

As dementia advances, patients face increasing threats to their independence and safety. Clinicians may be called on to address not only behavioral and psychological symptoms of dementia, such as agitation, hallucinations, and depression, but also risks of falling, fire hazards, driving safety, financial exploitation, medication nonadherence or refusal, refusal of care, hoarding, and firearm safety. If persons with dementia and their family members do not raise these issues themselves, clinicians should screen them for any concerns related to falling, driving, accidentally setting a fire, access to firearms, and other hazards around the home. Clinicians may need to collaborate with other health care professionals (e.g., social workers) in counseling persons with dementia and their family members and linking them to relevant resources in the community. These may be sensitive and emotionally challenging topics for patients and families and, in the case of addressing medication refusal, may also be ethically and clinically complex. Many of the screening items discussed in this chapter are included in the "Pre-evaluation Form" in the Appendix.

KEY POINTS

- To help reduce the risk of falls, the clinician should first identify and address risk factors (e.g., medications, orthostatic hypotension, vision loss). A physical therapist can help improve the patient's gait, strength, and balance and recommend an assistive device. A home-based or group exercise program should be recommended to the person with dementia. An in-home safety assessment by an occupational therapist may also be helpful. Engaging caregivers is critical in increasing home safety and in implementing an exercise program.

- A number of steps can be taken in the home to reduce the risk of fire and associated injury for persons with dementia and their family members, including restricting access to cooking equipment and addressing tobacco use. Persons with dementia who are still smoking should be encouraged to quit smoking and offered tobacco cessation treatment.

- Persons with moderate or severe dementia should not drive. Patients with MCI and mild dementia should be screened for safety concerns, should be encouraged to stop driving or undergo formal driving evaluation, and should seek alternate means of transportation. Family members may need support during potentially challenging discussions with their loved one.

- Financial incapacity can lead to an increased risk of financial abuse and exploitation. Clinicians should screen for financial incapacity, educate patients and families about reducing the risk of exploitation, and monitor for financial abuse.

- As dementia progresses, patients will need assistance from family members and other caregivers to ensure that they are taking their medications correctly. Caregiver education, pill boxes, blister packaging, and automated pill dispensers can be helpful. Dissolvable, liquid, or patch formulations should be considered for patients with swallowing difficulties.

- Medication refusal can be dangerous to the person with dementia and frustrating for caregivers. The reason for refusal should be identified (side effects, swallowing difficulties, paranoia, suicidal ideation) and addressed. Covert administration of medications may be ethically allowable in certain circumstances.
- Approaches to reducing refusal of assistance with ADLs include addressing pain, depression, delusions, and delirium; playing music during ADLs; and using a person-centered approach to bathing (namely, respecting privacy and promoting comfort).
- Refusing to eat or drink may indicate that the patient is in the final stage of dementia.
- Hoarding behavior is common among persons with dementia and can lead to serious medical and functional consequences. The following may be helpful: treating comorbid behavioral and psychological symptoms of dementia (e.g., depression, psychosis, obsessions, compulsions, impulsivity), psychotherapy, making use of organizations that can help people "dig out" of their homes, and referral to social service agencies.
- The most common suicide method among older adults is use of a firearm. Persons with moderate and severe dementia should not have access to a firearm. Clinicians should screen for depression, suicidal ideation, homicidal ideation, and paranoia when determining whether it is safe for persons with MCI or mild dementia to have access to a firearm. Clinicians should counsel persons with dementia and their family members regarding the risk of accidental or intentional injury.

RESOURCES FOR PATIENTS, FAMILIES, AND CAREGIVERS

Allen K: Refusing to Take Medications: Tips for the Alzheimer's Caregiver. Clarksburg, MD, Bright Focus Foundation, 2017. Available at: https://www.brightfocus.org/alzheimers/article/refusing-take-medications-tips-alzheimers-caregiver. This article provides a detailed description of how caregivers can help address medication refusal.

The Alzheimer's Store (https://www.alzstore.com/Default.asp) offers products to enhance home safety for patients with dementia and their family members. Examples of items include bed alarm sensors, automatic pill dispensers, door locks and alarms to address wandering, and wearable GPS locators.

Centers for Disease Control and Prevention: STEADI—Older Adult Fall Prevention. Atlanta, GA, Centers for Disease Control and Prevention, 2017. Available at: https://www.cdc.gov/steadi/index.html. This web page includes information for patients, caregivers, and clinicians regarding the Stopping Elderly Accidents, Deaths and Injuries (STEADI) program to reduce risk of falls.

Electrical Safety Foundation International: Home Fire Safety for Older Adults Safety Awareness Program Toolkit. Rosslyn, VA, Electrical Safety Foundation International, 2015. Available at: https://www.esfi.org/resource/home-fire-safety-for-older-adults-safety-awareness-program-toolkit-248. This web page lists a number of safety tips related to cooking, the kitchen, home heating, electrical safety, fire escape planning, and smoke alarm safety specifically for older adults. Many of these tips are applicable to persons with dementia and their family members.

HealthinAging.org: Aging & Health A to Z: Driving Safety for Older Adults. New York, Health in Aging Foundation, 2017. Available at: https://www.healthinaging.org/a-z-topic/driving-safety-older-adults. This web page provides links to a number of helpful documents, including tips for family members discussing with loved ones when it is time to stop driving and finding alternate means of transportation.

National Highway Traffic Safety Administration: How to Understand and Influence Older Drivers. Washington, DC, National Highway Traffic Safety Administration, 2018. Available at: https://www.nhtsa.gov/older-drivers/how-understand-and-influence-older-drivers. This web page provides comprehensive information to family members regarding collecting information about driving safety, having a conversation about driving concerns, and ensuring mobility for the person with dementia.

National Institute on Aging: Home Safety Checklist for Alzheimer's Disease. Bethesda, MD, National Institute on Aging, 2017. Available at: https://www.nia.nih.gov/health/home-safety-checklist-alzheimers-disease. This web page provides a comprehensive list of steps to take within the home to help keep persons with Alzheimer's disease and other causes of dementia safe. The list focuses on safety of outside approaches to the home and in individual rooms.

National Institute on Aging: Managing Medicines for a Person with Alzheimer's. Bethesda, MD, National Institute on Aging, 2017. Available at: https://www.nia.nih.gov/health/managing-medicines-person-alzheimers. This web page has a variety of tips for family members about being aware of what medications are being prescribed and about ensuring that medications are being taken safely.

National Institute on Aging: Managing Money Problems in Alzheimer's Disease. Bethesda, MD, National Institute on Aging, 2017. Available at: https://www.nia.nih.gov/health/managing-money-problems-alzheimers-disease. This web page presents information for family members about the signs of financial incapacity, steps that families can take to address financial incapacity, and guarding against scams.

REFERENCES

Allen K: Refusing to Take Medications: Tips for the Alzheimer's Caregiver. Bright Focus Foundation. Clarksburg, MD, BrightFocus Foundation, 2017. Available at: https://www.brightfocus.org/alzheimers/article/refusing-take-medications-tips-alzheimers-caregiver. Accessed August 9, 2018.

Alzheimer's Association: Home Safety. Chicago, IL, Alzheimer's Association, 2018a. Available at: https://www.alz.org/help-support/caregiving/safety/home-safety. Accessed August 8, 2018.

Alzheimer's Association: Medication Safety. Chicago, IL, Alzheimer's Association, 2018b. Available at: https://www.alz.org/help-support/caregiving/safety/medication-safety. Accessed August 9, 2018.

American Psychiatric Association: Diagnostic and Statistical Manual of Mental Disorders, 5th Edition. Arlington, VA, American Psychiatric Association, 2013

Aston L, Hilton A, Moutela T, et al: Exploring the evidence base for how people with dementia and their informal carers manage their medication in the community: a mixed studies review. BMC Geriatr 17(1):242–252, 2017 29047339

Ayers CR, Najmi S, Mayes TL, et al: Hoarding disorder in older adulthood. Am J Geriatr Psychiatry 23(4):416–422, 2015 24953872

Bennett JM, Chekaluk E, Batchelor J: Cognitive tests and determining fitness to drive in dementia: a systematic review. J Am Geriatr Soc 64(9):1904–1917, 2016 27253511

Betz ME, McCourt AD, Vernick JS, et al: Firearms and dementia: clinical considerations. Ann Intern Med 169(1):47–49, 2018 29801058

Bixby K, Davis JD, Ott BR: Comparing caregiver and clinician predictions of fitness to drive in people with Alzheimer's disease. Am J Occup Ther 69(3):1–7, 2015 25871601

Burnes D, Henderson CR Jr, Sheppard C, et al: Prevalence of financial fraud and scams among older adults in the United States: a systematic review and meta-analysis. Am J Public Health 107(8):e13–e21, 2017 28640686

Burton E, Cavalheri V, Adams R, et al: Effectiveness of exercise programs to reduce falls in older people with dementia living in the community: a systematic review and meta-analysis. Clin Interv Aging 10:421–434, 2015 25709416

Carter K, Monaghan S, O'Brien J, et al: Driving and dementia: a clinical decision pathway. Int J Geriatr Psychiatry 30(2):210–216, 2015 24865643

Cataldo JK, Glantz SA: Smoking cessation and Alzheimer's disease: facts, fallacies and promise. Expert Rev Neurother 10(5):629–631, 2010 20420482

Centers for Disease Control and Prevention: Family Caregivers: Prevent Your Loved Ones From Falling. Atlanta, GA, Centers for Disease Control and Prevention, 2017. Available at: https://www.cdc.gov/steadi/pdf/patient/customizable/Caregiver-Brochure-Final-Customizable-508.pdf. Accessed December 6, 2018.

Chaudhuri S, Thompson H, Demiris G: Fall detection devices and their use with older adults: a systematic review. J Geriatr Phys Ther 37(4):178–196, 2014 24406708

Electrical Safety Foundation International: Home Fire Safety for Older Adults Safety Awareness Program Toolkit. Rosslyn, VA, Electrical Safety Foundation International, 2015. Available at: https://www.esfi.org/resource/home-fire-safety-for-older-adults-safety-awareness-program-toolkit-248. Accessed August 8, 2018.

Elliott RA, Goeman D, Beanland C, Koch S: Ability of older people with dementia or cognitive impairment to manage medicine regimens: a narrative review. Curr Clin Pharmacol 10(3):213–221, 2015 26265487

Frank C, Misiaszek B: Approach to hoarding in family medicine: beyond reality television. Can Fam Physician 58(10):1087–1091, 2012 23064916

Gillespie LD, Robertson MC, Gillespie WJ, et al: Interventions for preventing falls in older people living in the community. Cochrane Database Syst Rev (9):CD007146, 2012 22972103

Haskins DR, Wick JY: Medication refusal: resident rights, administration dilemma. Consult Pharm 32(12):728–736, 2017 29467065

Huang Y, Britton J, Hubbard R, et al: Who receives prescriptions for smoking cessation medications? An association rule mining analysis using a large primary care database. Tob Control 22(4):274–279, 2013 22246781

Hung EK, McNiel DE, Binder RL: Covert medication in psychiatric emergencies: is it ever ethically permissible? J Am Acad Psychiatry Law 40(2):239–245, 2012 22635297

Ishii S, Streim JE, Saliba D: Potentially reversible resident factors associated with rejection of care behaviors. J Am Geriatr Soc 58(9):1693–1700, 2010 20863329

Iverson DJ, Gronseth GS, Reger MA, et al: Practice Parameter update: evaluation and management of driving risk in dementia: report of the Quality Standards Subcommittee of the American Academy of Neurology. Neurology 74(16):1316–1324, 2010 20860481

Konno R, Kang HS, Makimoto K: A best-evidence review of intervention studies for minimizing resistance-to-care behaviours for older adults with dementia in nursing homes. J Adv Nurs 70(10):2167–2180, 2014 24738712

Laver K, Dyer S, Whitehead C, et al: Interventions to delay functional decline in people with dementia: a systematic review of systematic reviews. BMJ Open 6(4):e010767, 2016 27121704

Lum HD, Flaten HK, Betz ME: Gun access and safety practices among older adults. Curr Gerontol Geriatr Res 2016:2980416, 2016 26949391

Marson DC: Clinical and ethical aspects of financial capacity in dementia: a commentary. Am J Geriatr Psychiatry 21(4):392–400, 2013 24078779

Marson DC, Sawrie SM, Snyder S, et al: Assessing financial capacity in patients with Alzheimer disease: a conceptual model and prototype instrument. Arch Neurol 57(6):877–884, 2000 10867786

Morris JC: The Clinical Dementia Rating (CDR): current version and scoring rules. Neurology 43(11):2412–2414, 1993 8232972

National Institute on Aging: Home Safety Checklist for Alzheimer's Disease. Bethesda, MD, National Institute on Aging, 2017a. Available at: https://www.nia.nih.gov/health/home-safety-checklist-alzheimers-disease. Accessed August 8, 2018.

National Institute on Aging: Managing Medicines for a Person with Alzheimer's. Bethesda, MD, National Institute on Aging, 2017b. Available at: https://www.nia.nih.gov/health/managing-medicines-person-alzheimers. Accessed August 9, 2018.

Peterson JC, Burnes DP, Caccamise PL, et al: Financial exploitation of older adults: a population-based prevalence study. J Gen Intern Med 29(12):1615–1623, 2014 25103121

Phelan EA, Mahoney JE, Voit JC, et al: Assessment and management of fall risk in primary care settings. Med Clin North Am 99(2):281–293, 2015 25700584

Pomidor A (ed): Clinician's Guide to Assessing and Counseling Older Drivers, 3rd Edition. (Report No DOT HS 812 228.) Washington, DC, National Highway Traffic Safety Administration, 2016

Rabins PV, Blacker D, Rovner BW, et al: American Psychiatric Association practice guideline for the treatment of patients with Alzheimer's disease and other dementias, second edition. Am J Psychiatry 164 (12 suppl):5–56, 2007

Rowe MA, Fehrenbach N: Injuries sustained by community-dwelling individuals with dementia. Clin Nurs Res 13(2):98–110, discussion 111–116, 2004 15104853

Royal College of Psychiatrists: College statement on covert administration of medicines. Psychiatr Bull 28(10):385–386, 2004

Sanders AE, Nininger J, Absher J, et al: Quality improvement in neurology: Dementia Management Quality Measurement Set update. Am J Psychiatry 174(5):493–498, 2017 28457155

Stout SH, Babulal GM, Ma C, et al: Driving cessation over a 24-year period: dementia severity and cerebrospinal fluid biomarkers. Alzheimers Dement 14(5):610–616, 2018 29328928

Young JM, Unger D: Covert administration of medication to persons with dementia: exploring ethical dimensions. J Clin Ethics 27(4):290–297, 2016 28001136

CHAPTER 7

ETHICAL AND LEGAL CONSIDERATIONS

Précis

Caring for persons with dementia in a humane and ethical way requires respecting their autonomy while simultaneously supporting their safety and welfare. The very nature of dementia threatens a person's autonomy and can lead to ethical conflicts as family members and clinicians step in to care for the person. In a medical setting, the primary ethical issue that arises in the care of persons with behavioral and psychological symptoms of dementia (BPSD) is impaired decisional capacity, requiring a clinician to assess decision-making capacity and address incapacity. Persons with BPSD are also at high risk of elder abuse, either through abuse, exploitation, neglect, or self-neglect. Clinicians have a key role in detecting elder abuse and have a legal obligation to report suspected elder abuse.

BACKGROUND: ETHICAL CARE OF THE PERSON WITH DEMENTIA

Ethically sound clinical care requires weighing principles that could come into conflict with each other. The principles of medical ethics include patient autonomy, patient welfare, and social justice (ABIM Foundation et al. 2002). The value of *autonomy* is foundational: We presuppose that people ought to be allowed to make decisions about their own lives. As such, *decisional capacity*, as well as the ability to provide *informed consent*, arises from one's autonomy. Autonomy encompasses not only the ability to make decisions but also the abilities to maintain a sense of self, to express one's values, and to engage in important relationships (Nuffield Council on Bioethics 2009). Supporting the *welfare* of patients involves both beneficence, wherein

225

a clinician performs or recommends action that will improve the patient's health, and nonmaleficence, wherein clinicians are prohibited from acting in ways that could harm patients—in other words, "first, do no harm." Advocating for *social justice* involves the imperative to address inequalities that affect the health of individuals and the public.

Ethical conflicts can arise in the care of persons with dementia and in their relationship with their caregivers. The cognitive, emotional, behavioral, and functional impairments of dementia impinge on the person's ability to form new memories and recall old ones, to rationally manipulate information, to understand and appreciate his or her situation, to make and express choices about his or her welfare, and even to maintain a coherent sense of self (Walaszek 2011). Loss of these capacities leads to the core ethical issue in the care of persons with BPSD.

Underpinning the process of addressing ethical conflicts in dementia care is the belief that "with good care and support, people with dementia can expect to have a good quality of life throughout the course of their illness" (Nuffield Council on Bioethics 2009, p. 21). Furthermore, "the person with dementia remains the same, equally valued, person throughout the course of their illness, regardless of the extent of the changes in their cognitive and other functions" (Nuffield Council on Bioethics 2009, p. 21).

The next section of this chapter focuses on the topic of decisional capacity in persons with BPSD; the discussion includes assessment of capacity and addressing of incapacity. Persons with dementia are also at risk of being abused or exploited; this is explored in the section "Protecting the Vulnerable Elder With Dementia." The final section covers ethical issues that arise in the provision of psychiatric care and palliative care to persons with BPSD.

Other important ethical issues in the care of persons with dementia include capacity to participate in research, end-of-life care (including artificial nutrition and hydration), physician-assisted suicide and euthanasia, addressing stigma associated with the diagnosis of dementia, and ensuring that persons with dementia receive just and equitable health care. These topics are beyond the scope of this book; interested readers are referred to a review such as the one by Gauthier et al. (2013).

DECISIONAL CAPACITY AND OTHER CAPACITIES

For individuals to have the capacity to make a decision (i.e., *decisional capacity*), they must understand the information relevant to that decision, must appreciate that the decision is relevant to them, must be able to reason (i.e., logically manipulate information), and must be able to express a choice (Roberts and Dyer 2004). Although a diagnosis of dementia in and of itself does not necessarily mean that a person cannot make decisions about his or her health and welfare, the ability to make decisions decreases markedly over the course of the illness (Walaszek 2011). This is especially true in moderate and severe stages of dementia, which is when especially troubling BPSD such as agitation, psychosis, and apathy tend to arise.

A clinician caring for a person with dementia must seek consent from that person before providing a specific intervention or medical care in general. Being able to provide informed consent requires that the person has relevant information available, can make and express a free choice without coercion (referred to as *voluntarism*), and has decisional capacity (Roberts 2002). Unfortunately, a person with dementia—and especially with BPSD—may face significant barriers to voluntarism, including cognitive impairment (especially amnesia, executive dysfunction, and lack of insight), agitation, delusions, apathy, depression (including hopelessness), pressure or coercion by family members or other caregivers, and abuse or exploitation (Roberts 2002). Figure 7–1 summarizes the relationships among voluntarism, decisional capacity, and informed consent.

Of course, health care decisions are not the only decisions that persons with dementia must make. To function independently, they must make choices about daily life (e.g., what to eat, what to wear, when to bathe, how to take medications), about their finances, about driving, about whether and with whom to have sexual relations, about voting, and about future planning (e.g., naming a power of attorney [POA] and executing a will). The cognitive, emotional, and behavioral impairments associated with dementia may affect these various capacities. I discuss driving capacity and financial capacity in Chapter 6. See Walaszek (2009) for a detailed discussion of other capacities, including their assessment. Note that *capacity* is different from *competence*, which is a legal determination about the person's ability to manage his or her affairs.

Assessing Capacity

When the clinician is assessing and managing BPSD, the question of medical decision-making capacity is likely to arise at some point. The clinician may need to assess whether the person with BPSD is able to provide informed consent to the assessment and management of BPSD. In some cases, the answer may be obvious. For example, a person with advanced dementia who requires assistance in most activities of daily living most likely will not be able to consent to be treated for agitation with an antipsychotic;

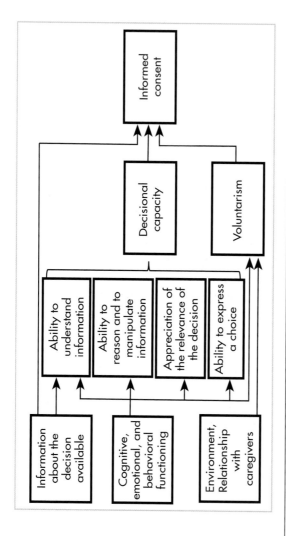

FIGURE 7–1.   Model of the ability of persons with behavioral and psychological symptoms of dementia (BPSD) to consent to treatment.

To provide informed consent, a person must have relevant information available, must have decisional capacity, and should not face barriers to voluntarism. Decisional capacity in turn requires having the ability to understand information, the ability to reason, appreciation of the relevance of the decision, and the ability to express a choice. A person with BPSD may have cognitive, emotional, and behavioral impairments that affect either voluntarism or one or more of the four elements of decisional capacity. Voluntarism also depends on being free from coercion, abuse, and exploitation, which in turn depends on the environment and relationship with caregivers.

Source.   Roberts 2002; Roberts and Dyer 2004.

conversely, a person with mild cognitive impairment likely retains the capacity to consent to be treated for depression with problem-solving psychotherapy. I suspect that many clinically challenging situations rest in the gray area between these two extremes and so require more comprehensive assessment of capacity.

In general, the threshold of capacity required to consent to treatment is higher when the risks of treatment are relatively high or when the benefits are relatively low; this is referred to as a "sliding scale" of capacity (Drane 1984). Potential benefits of treatment include reducing frequency and severity of symptoms, improving quality of life, and reducing the chance of harm; potential risks include physical side effects and threats to autonomy and voluntarism. Risks and benefits of interventions can be estimated based on the discussion in Chapter 5.

The threshold of capacity also depends on whether the patient is accepting or refusing a treatment. For example, the threshold for accepting a low-risk, high-benefit intervention (e.g., phlebotomy to determine if an electrolyte disturbance could be contributing to BPSD) is low, whereas the threshold for refusing such an intervention is high.

Usually, medical decision-making capacity refers to a specific decision. Patients may retain the capacity to provide consent for some medical interventions but not others. However, impairment that affects making one medical decision should raise the question about whether the patient is more globally impaired—that is, unable to make *any* medical decisions. Determining whether a person with dementia lacks the capacity to make medical decisions in general entails a more in-depth assessment, which is outside the scope of this chapter.

To assess a patient's capacity to consent to or refuse an intervention, the clinician asks a series of questions meant to elicit the patient's understanding, appreciation, reasoning, and ability to express a choice (Karlawish 2008; Moye et al. 2007; Palmer and Harmell 2016; Walaszek 2009).

- *Understanding* refers to the ability of the person to comprehend information about the proposed treatment, including the risks and benefits of treatment, alternatives to treatment, and the risks and benefits of no treatment. A clinician can assess understanding by presenting information about the recommended treatment and then asking the patient to repeat the information in his or her own words.
- *Appreciation* refers to the ability of the person to apply the information to his or her own particular situation. The clinician can assess this by probing the patient's beliefs about his or her diagnosis and about the benefit

he or she personally can expect to get from treatment. A person with dementia who is unaware of his or her own cognitive impairment might be able to understand and reason but may not appreciate that the decision to be made is about him or her personally.

- *Reasoning* refers to the ability of the person with dementia to manipulate information logically and consistently. The clinician asks the patient to state the consequences, both positive and negative, of deciding for or against a treatment and, if relevant, to compare options.

- *Expressing a choice* refers to whether a person with dementia, having made a decision, can inform others of this decision. Some have argued (and I concur) that the patient must express a *consistent* choice; therefore, using this standard, a patient with delirium who alternately agrees to and refuses an intervention would not have capacity.

The Aid to Capacity Evaluation (ACE) operationalizes this process (Etchells et al. 1999; also available at www.jcb.utoronto.ca/tools/documents/ace.pdf). In addition to covering the four areas just listed, the ACE instructs the clinician to assess for paranoia (e.g., "Do you think anyone is trying to hurt/harm you?") and for depression (e.g., "Do you have any hope for the future?") as symptoms potentially affecting decisional capacity. If the patient is found to lack capacity, these questions can identify potentially reversible causes of incapacity. The ACE is also a reminder that, because people are presumed capable, a clinician who is uncertain about a person's decisional capacity should err on the side of saying that the person has decisional capacity.

Bedside tests may serve as adjuncts to capacity evaluation but do not replace the process described here. The Mini-Mental State Examination (MMSE) is the bedside cognitive test most studied with respect to capacity: a score greater than 24 is predictive of capacity, whereas a score lower than 18 is predictive of incapacity (Kim et al. 2002). I would argue that bedside testing may help the clinician get a general idea about the patient's capacity—a normal or nearly normal result suggests that the patient has capacity, whereas a grossly abnormal result suggests that the patient does not have capacity—but a formal assessment is ultimately necessary. Similarly, the stage of dementia severity may help predict capacity: patients with mild cognitive impairment (Clinical Dementia Rating [CDR] of 0.5) are most likely to retain capacity, those with mild dementia (CDR of 1) are less likely to have capacity, and those with moderate or severe dementia (CDR of 2 or 3) are unlikely to have capacity (Karlawish et al. 2002). BPSD themselves, specifically delusions and apathy, may affect decisional capacity

(Bertrand et al. 2017). Most of the research on capacity has involved Alzheimer's disease; it is unclear how much the etiology of dementia affects capacity, though it stands to reason that persons with frontotemporal dementia are more likely to have impaired capacity early in the course of illness due to executive dysfunction and problems with judgment.

See Table 7–1 for a summary of the assessment of the capacity of a person with BPSD to consent to or to refuse to consent to an intervention, and see Case Example 7–1 for a discussion involving one of the more common capacity scenarios in the care of patients with BPSD: refusal of an intervention that is likely to benefit the patient and to address safety concerns.

Case Example 7–1: "I'm Pretty Sure He Won't Take Any New Medications."

Mr. Robinson is an 81-year-old man with Alzheimer's disease who moved into an assisted living facility 2 years ago, after the death of his wife, who had been his primary caregiver. He has dementia of moderate severity and requires assistance with meals and medications and sometimes needs reminders to complete personal hygiene tasks. Mr. Robinson has hypertension, dyslipidemia, and diabetes mellitus and intermittently refuses to take medications for these conditions. He has historically distrusted doctors and takes prescribed medications grudgingly. He carefully reviews each pill he is given by the medical assistant and gets upset when a new medication appears.

Over the past 3 months, Mr. Robinson has become physically aggressive with the caregiving staff and, on one occasion, with another resident of the facility. The staff has worked hard but without much success to identify triggers and a pattern for the behavior. Redirection and validation have been partially effective, but he still has daily "explosions" of anger and agitation, with the most recent episode resulting in injury to a caregiver whose arm he grabbed. The director of nursing asks Mr. Robinson's doctor to prescribe a medication to address agitation but is also skeptical that Mr. Robinson will accept a new medication.

Mr. Robinson's doctor carefully reviews the history and interviews the patient. Although Mr. Robinson is generally calm throughout the interview, he is intermittently irritable and guarded. Screening for BPSD reveals that Mr. Robinson experiences some paranoia, especially about food ("Who knows what they put in there to make me sick?") and medications ("You're going to get rich giving me all those pills"). Mr. Robinson's doctor, carefully weighing the risks and benefits, recommends a trial of risperidone to address paranoia and physical aggression that could pose a danger to himself and others. Mr. Robinson, as the director of nursing guessed he would, refuses this medication.

Mr. Robinson's doctor wonders, given the severity of the patient's dementia, whether he has the capacity to refuse to consent to this intervention. Therefore, the doctor performs a decisional capacity evaluation. The

TABLE 7–1. Determining whether a patient has capacity to consent to or to refuse treatment for behavioral and psychological symptoms of dementia (BPSD)

Baseline estimate of capacity	Patient is more likely to have capacity if
	MMSE > 24
	Mild cognitive impairment (CDR = 0.5)
	Patient is less likely to have capacity if
	MMSE < 18
	Moderate or severe dementia (CDR = 2–3)
	Etiology of dementia is frontotemporal dementia
Threshold of capacity required	To consent to treatment
	Higher threshold is required for low-benefit, high-risk interventions
	Lower threshold is required for high-benefit, low-risk interventions
	To refuse treatment
	Higher threshold is required for high-benefit, low-risk interventions
	Lower threshold is required for low-benefit, high-risk interventions
Formal capacity assessment	The patient has capacity to accept or refuse treatment if he or she demonstrates understanding, appreciation, reasoning, *and* ability to consistently express a choice (all four elements of decisional capacity) at the threshold determined above.
	Otherwise, the patient does not have capacity.
Potentially reversible causes of incapacity	If the patient does not have capacity, assess for and address the following:
	Depression or hopelessness
	Apathy
	Psychosis
	Delirium
	Medications causing cognitive impairment
	Vision or hearing loss
	Lack of knowledge regarding dementia or BPSD

Note. CDR = Clinical Dementia Rating instrument; MMSE = Mini-Mental State Examination.

doctor explains the situation to Mr. Robinson, including his diagnosis (Alzheimer's disease), the indication for risperidone (agitation), the benefits and risks (including mortality), and the alternatives (continued nonpharmacological interventions). Mr. Robinson has trouble restating the details in his own terms and needs to have the information repeated. Mr. Robinson denies that he has Alzheimer's disease and does not recall having been agitated, so he does not see why this medication would be prescribed to him. He continues to decline a trial of risperidone. Given Mr. Robinson's lack of understanding and appreciation, the doctor determines that Mr. Robinson lacks decisional capacity. Paperwork in Mr. Robinson's chart indicates that his health care power of attorney is his son, who lives in a neighboring suburb; Mr. Robinson's doctor calls his son to discuss this medical decision.

Preparing for Incapacity

The process of determining capacity just described leads to a dichotomous outcome: namely, whether or not a person has decisional capacity. This result ignores that many persons with dementia are able to make medical decisions with the support of family members; in fact, bioethicists have argued strongly for engaging the family members of persons with dementia in making medical decisions (Nuffield Council on Bioethics 2009). However, as far as I know, there are no jurisdictions with legal procedures to officially enable this sort of shared decision making among persons with dementia, their family members, and their treatment providers; therefore, patients and families must rely on informal mechanisms instead (Kapp 2002). For example, a person with dementia who has been incapacitated might, with appropriate support, be able to participate in a decision-making process with the proxy, who "officially" makes the decision.

Ideally, as discussed in the section "Planning for the Future and Legal Considerations" in Chapter 2, a person with dementia will have designated a health care POA prior to losing the capacity to make medical decisions. Then, if and when the person with dementia becomes incapacitated, the POA assumes responsibility for these decisions. In reality, most persons with dementia have not designated a health care POA. If a patient retains the capacity to designate a health care POA but has lost other medical decision-making capacity, it is ethically permissible to ask a patient to designate a health care POA and then to "activate" the POA. This follows from the notion that different decisions require different levels of capacity. For example, a person with dementia who has had a long-standing and supportive relationship with his or her spouse or partner for many years does not require a terribly high threshold for decisional capacity to designate this person as his or her POA. On the other hand, naming a long-lost relative whom the person with dementia has not seen for many years requires a higher threshold for capacity.

Clinicians caring for persons with BPSD are in a unique position to address the issue of incapacity because they are probably more likely than most other clinicians to encounter patients without the capacity to make medical decisions. Therefore, I recommend 1) maintaining a high index of suspicion for incapacity, 2) conducting a capacity assessment whenever incapacity is suspected, 3) engaging trusted family members and caregivers in care, and 4) strongly recommending that all persons with dementia formally select a health care POA. Clinicians should be aware of local laws and regulations relevant to the selection of a health care POA and to "activation" of the POA.

Addressing Incapacity

When a person with dementia is found to lack the capacity to make medical decisions, a surrogate will need to assume responsibility for making such decisions. If the person with dementia has designated a health care POA, that person becomes the proxy decision maker. If not, then the legal next of kin becomes the proxy decision maker. In some cases, a guardian may need to be selected via a legal process.

Proxy (or surrogate) decision makers can follow one or both standards for determining the right course of action for a person with dementia: *best interest* or *substituted judgment* (Gutheil and Appelbaum 2000). Proxies who make medical decisions based on what they believe is in the best interest of a person with dementia, weighing risks and benefits themselves, are using the best interest standard. Proxies who make a decision based on the choice they think a person with dementia would have made (based on informal discussion prior to the person losing capacity, or on an understanding of the person's values and desires, or on the wishes expressed in an advance directive) are using the substituted judgment standard. A hybrid approach has been recommended, wherein substituted judgment is used when the person's wishes are clear, and otherwise, best interest is used (Gutheil and Appelbaum 2000).

As presented in Table 7–1, clinicians should try to identify and address reversible causes of incapacity, including depression, hopelessness, apathy, psychosis, delirium, medication side effect, hearing loss, and vision loss (Walaszek 2009). If possible, clinicians should attempt to use cognitive and educational strategies to restore capacity—for example, teaching the patient about dementia and BPSD. These interventions may help eventually restore capacity, especially in the case of delirium, which may result in only temporary incapacity.

Of course, if a patient refuses a medication and is deemed not to have capacity to refuse the medication, there remains the issue of how to administer the medication. One option is the covert administration of medication, discussed in the section "Adherence to Medications" in Chapter 6. Another option could be parenteral administration, but this is both impractical (most medications do not have parenteral forms, let alone long-acting formulations such as Risperdal Consta) and potentially inhumane.

A detailed discussion of guardianship is beyond the scope of this book, so I review the topic briefly here. A court may declare a person who is unable to make everyday decisions, manage his or her affairs, and live independently, to be *incompetent*. (Capacity may be a medical decision; competency is always a legal decision.) The court then appoints a guardian (or conservator) to manage the affairs of the person deemed incompetent. Clinicians will then need to seek consent for medical treatment from the guardian; therefore, clinicians should make themselves familiar with local laws and regulations governing guardianship and the rights of the person declared incompetent. Readers interested in learning more about clinicians' evaluation of patients for guardianship are referred to the review by Moye et al. (2007).

PROTECTING THE VULNERABLE ELDER WITH DEMENTIA

As noted in the discussion in Chapter 2, the prevalence of elder abuse among older adults in general is 11% and among those with dementia is up to 62%; cognitive impairment is among the most consistently reported risk factors for elder abuse (Alosa Health 2017; Dong et al. 2014). With respect to specific types of abuse, the 1-year prevalence among older adults of emotional abuse is 4.6%, physical abuse 1.6%, neglect (including self-neglect) 5.1%, and financial mistreatment by family 5.2% (Acierno et al. 2010). Abuse is underreported by older adults, likely because of cognitive impairment, fear of retaliation, and fear of losing the support of their family (Dong et al. 2014).

Clinicians should maintain a high index of suspicion that any person with dementia could be a victim of elder abuse, especially if one or more of the following risk factors are present: age older than 80, female sex, black or Hispanic ethnicity, lower income, three or more medical conditions, MMSE score less than 23, impaired physical functioning, depression, social isolation, and violent behavior on the part of the patient (Alosa Health 2017). Unfortunately, physicians are relatively unlikely to report elder abuse, accounting for only 1.4% of reporters; possible reasons include feeling that abuse could not be proved, signs of abuse were subtle, the patient denied being mistreated, being unsure of reporting procedures and resources, and fear of harming the relationship with the patient (Alosa Health 2017).

The Elder Abuse Suspicion Index (EASI; Table 2–3 in Chapter 2) has modest sensitivity and specificity for detecting elder abuse among community-dwelling elders (Yaffe et al. 2008); see Table 2–3 and accompanying text in Chapter 2 for more details. The U.S. Centers for Medicare and Medicaid Services recommends screening for abuse with the Vulnerability to Abuse Screening Scale (VASS) or the Hwalek-Sengstock Elder Abuse Screening Test (H-S/EAST), though they also have high false-negative rates and do not probe subtypes of elder abuse (both are reproduced in Dong 2015). None of these tools have been validated in people with cognitive impairment. The Elder Abuse Decision Support System (EADSS)—Adult Mistreatment Assessment Short Form is more comprehensive and has been validated in a large sample of subjects drawn from elder abuse investigations, but it is lengthy (36 questions) and intended for use by adult protective services (APS) workers (Beach et al. 2017). With respect to screening tools, my advice to clinicians is to use the EASI and to keep in mind the possibility of false-negative scores—therefore, if suspicion is high, further questioning may be necessary. Questions about abuse and neglect should be asked of the patient without the presence of caregivers.

Clinicians must learn their local laws regarding the reporting of elder abuse. In general, clinicians must report suspected elder abuse to the appropriate local officials, such as an APS agency. A situation involving suspected elder abuse of a person without decisional capacity must be reported. A person with decisional capacity may decline assistance or intervention from the clinician or APS; in such cases, there should be close monitoring and, if relevant, another recommendation for intervention. The clinician must balance the autonomy of the patient, the welfare of the patient, the need to maintain a safe and healthy environment, and the integrity of the family unit.

See Table 7–2 for a summary regarding identifying elder abuse in persons with BPSD.

Self-Neglect

A person with dementia who is responsible for his or her own care demonstrates *self-neglect* when he or she fails to obtain adequate care, including food, shelter, clothing, medical care, dental care, and mental health care. A not uncommon scenario is for individuals with dementia who live alone to

TABLE 7–2.	Identifying elder abuse in persons with behavioral and psychological symptoms of dementia (BPSD)

1. Maintain a high index of suspicion because patients with dementia (and especially BPSD) are at risk of elder abuse.

2. Consider screening for elder abuse using a tool such as the Elder Abuse Suspicion Index (see Table 2–3).

3. Watch for signs of abuse or neglect.

   a. Medication nonadherence[a]

   b. Poor hygiene[a]

   c. Lack of needed medical equipment

   d. Malnourishment[a] or dehydration

   e. Physical signs of abuse or neglect: bruises,[a] welts, lacerations,[a] fractures, decubitus ulcers

   f. Apprehension of or withdrawal from caregivers

   g. Caregiver being demeaning to person with dementia

   h. Refusing to let caregivers or social services staff into the home

4. Ask about abuse or neglect.

   a. Have you been hit, kicked, punched, or slapped?[a]

   b. Have you been handled roughly, pushed, shoved, grabbed, or shaken?[a]

   c. Have you been physically injured in some other way?[a]

   d. Have you been called unkind names, put down, or made to feel like a child?[a]

   e. Have you been manipulated, controlled, or lied to by your caregiver?[a]

   f. Are you afraid of your caregiver or anyone else?[a]

   g. Have you not been allowed to speak for yourself?

   h. Have you been threatened with gestures such as fist shaking?

   i. Have you been forced into sexual activities?[a]

   j. Have you been otherwise threatened or not supported?

5. Report suspect cases to appropriate authorities.

   a. If patient is in imminent danger, call police or emergency medical services for immediate help.

   b. If patient is not in imminent danger and lacks decisional capacity, refer to adult protective services or comparable agency for investigation.

   c. If patient has decisional capacity and is willing to accept services, refer to adult protective services.

   d. If patient has decisional capacity but refuses services, monitor situation closely, offer support, and recommend referral again if indicated.

[a]Also covered to some extent in the Elder Abuse Suspicion Index (see Table 2–3 in Chapter 2).

become increasingly unable to care for themselves as dementia progresses. (It would be considered neglect rather than self-neglect if another responsible adult were living in the household.) In fact, self-neglect is the most common reason for referral to APS and is associated with high mortality (Dong et al. 2014).

Clinicians should be vigilant for signs of self-neglect such as medication nonadherence (which I consider a subtle early sign of self-neglect), poor hygiene (e.g., noticeable body odor, dirty clothing, long and dirty fingernails), a lack of needed medical equipment (e.g., eyeglasses, hearing aids, dentures, walker, wheelchair), malnourishment, and dehydration (Beach et al. 2017). (Note that poverty could account for some of these findings as well.) An in-home assessment, conducted by occupational therapists, nurses, or social workers, can help uncover self-neglect. Persons with self-neglect may come to clinical attention because of concern that they are depressed or because they are not allowing family members, health care professionals, or social services staff into their homes. Clinicians should consider the possibility that depression, apathy, anxiety, paranoia, or medication side effects are contributing to self-neglect and address those appropriately. Following local laws, clinicians should report suspected self-neglect to appropriate authorities.

Ultimately, a person with dementia and self-neglect may need to accept in-home services or move to a higher level of care—a reduction in autonomy in favor of the person's well-being. This process may be legally complex, requiring the appointment of a guardian.

Neglect and Abuse

Neglect reflects a failure on the part of a caregiver to try to obtain appropriate care, services, or supervision for the person with dementia (specifically, food, clothing, shelter, medical care, and mental health care). Abuse includes a wide range of problematic behaviors perpetrated by a caregiver toward a patient with dementia: physical abuse, emotional abuse, sexual abuse, treatment without consent (e.g., giving medications to a person without his or her knowledge—though in certain circumstances this may be ethically allowable, as discussed in the section "Adherence to Medications" in Chapter 6), and unreasonable confinement or restraint (e.g., locking a person with dementia in his or her room). Emotional abuse can involve verbal assaults, threats of maltreatment, harassment, intimidation, or compelling the person with dementia to act in a way opposed to his or her wishes (Beach et al. 2017).

Clinicians caring for persons with BPSD should maintain an especially high index of suspicion for abuse and neglect. In addition to being vigilant for the signs listed in the prior section on self-neglect (poor hygiene, lack of medical equipment, dehydration, malnourishment), clinicians should be mindful of physical signs of abuse or neglect (bruises, welts, lacerations, fractures, decubitus ulcers). In the presence of a caregiver, the person with dementia may appear apprehensive or withdrawn, or the caregiver may talk over or demean the person with dementia. In the absence of the caregiver, the clinician suspecting abuse should ask the person with dementia if he or she has been hit, kicked, punched, or slapped; handled roughly, pushed, shoved, grabbed, or shaken; physically injured in some other way; called unkind names, put down, or made to feel like a child; manipulated, controlled, or lied to by the caregiver; afraid of the caregiver; not allowed to speak for themselves; threatened with gestures such as fist shaking; forced into sexual activities; or otherwise threatened or unsupported (Beach et al. 2017). These can be very challenging conversations because the person with dementia may not recall instances of abuse or neglect, may be unwilling to "talk out of turn" about his or her family members or may be worried about getting them in trouble, may confabulate, or may be paranoid (and thereby make false accusations).

Ultimately, investigation by local authorities may be the only way to determine exactly what is going on and how best to help the person with dementia. Clinicians must report suspected abuse or neglect to local authorities or, if the person with dementia is in immediate danger, must call police or activate emergency medical services.

Financial Abuse

Most persons with mild dementia and almost all with moderate or severe dementia have problems managing their finances. Financial fraud and scams targeting older adults are common. and persons with dementia may be especially vulnerable. They may also be exploited by their own family members—behavior that constitutes elder abuse and that may be illegal. Examples of financial abuse or exploitation include obtaining money or property by deception, coercion, or theft; failure or neglect of the financial agent to fulfill financial responsibilities; and unauthorized use of documents or identity. See the section "Financial Incapacity and Risk of Exploitation" in Chapter 6 for further discussion. Case Example 7–2 presents the case of a person with dementia at risk of elder abuse.

Case Example 7–2: "She Won't Get Help and Is Getting Sicker and Sicker. I Think She's Depressed."

Mrs. Diaz is an 86-year-old widow with Parkinson disease dementia who lives alone. Her neighbors have become concerned about her because they rarely see her leave the house, and they are not sure she is getting enough to eat; when they briefly see her standing on her front stoop, they note that her clothes are unkempt and that she appears to have lost weight. She has several nieces and nephews but has not allowed any of them into her home recently. A local social worker has become involved and discovered that Mrs. Diaz's utilities are about to be turned off because she has not paid bills in several months. The social worker convinces Mrs. Diaz to be evaluated by her primary care provider.

Prior to the examination, the social worker pulls the primary care provider aside and says, "She won't get help and is getting sicker and sicker. I think she's depressed." Mrs. Diaz does in fact appear to be sullen and withdrawn. She is also wearing stained clothing and is faintly malodorous. She has a marked resting tremor involving her right arm, and she shuffles when she walks. Mrs. Diaz's blood pressure, formerly under control with lisinopril, is high today at 180/90. She weighs 30 pounds less than she had at her annual physical examination 6 months earlier. She is unable to provide much history herself but does vaguely refer to "bad guys" breaking into her home; it is unclear if this is paranoid ideation, visual hallucination, or both. She endorses feeling sad and wondering, "What is the point?" She denies suicidal ideation. She does not recall the names of her medications (lisinopril, carbidopa-levodopa, lovastatin, galantamine) or why she is taking them. She scores a 12 out of 30 on the Montreal Cognitive Assessment, down from 15 six months ago.

The primary care provider agrees that Mrs. Diaz may be depressed and is also concerned about the possibility of elder abuse, namely self-neglect. An antidepressant is recommended, and she consents, though the primary care provider is not certain that the patient will remember to take the medication. A referral to APS is recommended, but Mrs. Diaz refuses. Because it appears that she lacks the capacity to refuse this referral, the primary care provider contacts APS and requests an elder abuse investigation, which will hopefully lead to greater support and services for Mrs. Diaz.

ETHICAL CONSIDERATIONS IN THE PRESCRIPTION OF PSYCHOTROPIC MEDICATIONS AND IN PSYCHIATRIC HOSPITALIZATION

At first blush, the prescription of antipsychotic medications to older adults with dementia may seem to be a violation of the principle of nonmaleficence—after all, antipsychotic medications are associated with a higher risk of mortality. Furthermore, patients who are candidates for treatment with antipsychotic medications are unlikely, given the severity of their dementia and the nature of their BPSD, to be able to consent to such treatment. It has been argued that prescribing antipsychotic medications is ethically permissible as long as the purpose is to reduce the distress of the person with dementia and as long as no treatable physical or environmental causes have been found (Treloar et al. 2010). The clinician thereby assumes a palliative care approach—alleviating distress when life expectancy is short. My own experience is that most families, following a thorough discussion of risks, benefits, and alternatives, consent to this treatment that may shorten life as long as it reduces the distress their loved one is experiencing.

A slightly more nuanced issue is whether psychotropic medications can be administered to a person who lacks capacity to consent to or to refuse treatment. In some jurisdictions, psychotropic medications can be administered to someone against his or her will only in an emergency or if the patient meets the local criteria for involuntary psychiatric treatment (which typically requires the presence of a treatable mental illness and the potential for danger to self or others). A similar issue arises when patients with BPSD require admission to an inpatient unit, either a general psychiatric unit or a special care unit. Presumably, a person with BPSD who has capacity to consent to inpatient psychiatric care ought to be able to be admitted without controversy. On the other hand, when a person with BPSD lacks the capacity to consent to inpatient treatment, the proper course of action is less clear: it appears that some practitioners believe than an activated health care POA may be sufficient to admit the person, whereas others believe that this can only happen via the involuntary commitment process (Rissmiller et al. 2001); some jurisdictions prohibit the use of an activated POA to admit a person against his or her will (Walaszek 2009). Clinicians may wish to receive ethical or legal consultation in such situations.

SUMMARY: DOING THE RIGHT THING IN THE CARE OF A PERSON WITH DEMENTIA

We want to do what is best for our patients with BPSD. Doing the right thing may not be straightforward, however, because persons with dementia progressively lose their capacity to make decisions, may become targets of abuse and exploitation, may refuse interventions that appear to be in their best interests, may come into conflict with family members and other caregivers, and can be prescribed medications with a high potential for harm. Following the evidence-based recommendations presented over the course of this book and carefully weighing the ethical principles of respecting patients' autonomy and promoting their welfare will usually lead to the best outcomes for our patients and their family members.

KEY POINTS

- The principles of medical ethics include respecting each person's autonomy, supporting the person's welfare through beneficence and nonmaleficence ("first, do no harm"), and promoting social justice.

- For a medical intervention to take place, a person must provide informed consent. *Informed consent* means that the patient must have relevant information available, must have decisional capacity, and should not face barriers to voluntarism (i.e., is able to act without coercion).

- In turn, *decisional capacity* requires that the person can understand relevant information, logically manipulate information, appreciate that the situation applies to him or her, and consistently express a choice.

- When a person lacks decisional capacity and is unable to provide informed consent, a proxy must then make the decision. The proxy may be a legal next of kin, activated health care POA, or legally appointed guardian.

- A proxy decision maker may act in a way reflective of the patient's past wishes and values ("substituted judgment"), or may decide based on his or her own review of the risks and benefits ("best interest"), or may use a blend of the two approaches.

- Because persons with BPSD are at particularly high risk of developing incapacity (either because of BPSD themselves or because of the severity of dementia), clinicians should recommend that these persons identify their health care POA (and make other legal provisions) sooner rather than later.

- Rates of elder abuse are high among persons with BPSD. Clinicians are well positioned to identify self-neglect, neglect, abuse, and financial exploitation and should consider using a screening tool to help identify patients at risk of elder abuse. Clinicians must report suspected cases of elder abuse in accordance with local laws.

- Clinicians should consider the ethical issues associated with the prescription of antipsychotic medications to patients with BPSD and the possible legal issues associated with psychiatric hospitalization for patients with BPSD.

RESOURCES FOR PATIENTS, FAMILIES, AND CAREGIVERS

Alosa Health: Elder Abuse and Dementia. Boston, MA, Alosa Health, 2017. Available at: https://alosahealth.org/clinical-modules/elder-abuse. This well-written and visually appealing brochure informs older adults and their families regarding steps they can take to stay free of abuse and exploitation, red flags to watch for, and support that is available in case there is a concern. Alosa Health also instructs physicians in the academic detailing model of medical education, which involves content experts coming into clinical settings to educate practitioners.

REFERENCES

ABIM Foundation, ACP-ASIM Foundation, European Federation of Internal Medicine: Medical professionalism in the new millennium: a physician charter. Ann Intern Med 136(3):243–246, 2002 11827500

Acierno R, Hernandez MA, Amstadter AB, et al: Prevalence and correlates of emotional, physical, sexual, and financial abuse and potential neglect in the United States: the National Elder Mistreatment Study. Am J Public Health 100(2):292–297, 2010 20019303

Alosa Health: Caring for Vulnerable Elders: Addressing Elder Abuse, Managing Dementia, Supporting Caregivers. Boston, MA, Alosa Health, 2017 Available at: http://alosahealth.org/wp-content/uploads/2018/11/Elder_Abuse_EvDoc_Final.pdf. Accessed December 10, 2018.

Beach SR, Liu P-J, DeLiema M, et al: Development of short-form measures to assess four types of elder mistreatment: findings from an evidence-based study of APS elder abuse substantiation decisions. J Elder Abuse Negl 29(4):229–253, 2017 28590799

Bertrand E, van Duinkerken E, Landeira-Fernandez J, et al: Behavioral and psychological symptoms impact clinical competence in Alzheimer's disease. Front Aging Neurosci 9:182, 2017 28670272

Dong X: Screening for elder abuse in healthcare settings: why should we care, and is it a missed quality indicator? J Am Geriatr Soc 63(8):1686–1688, 2015 26277299

Dong X, Chen R, Simon MA: Elder abuse and dementia: a review of the research and health policy. Health Aff (Millwood) 33(4):642–649, 2014 24711326

Drane JF: Competency to give an informed consent: a model for making clinical assessments. JAMA 252(7):925–927, 1984 6748193

Etchells E, Darzins P, Silberfeld M, et al: Assessment of patient capacity to consent to treatment. J Gen Intern Med 14(1):27–34, 1999 9893088

Gauthier S, Leuzy A, Racine E, et al: Diagnosis and management of Alzheimer's disease: past, present and future ethical issues. Prog Neurobiol 110:102–113, 2013 23578568

Gutheil TG, Appelbaum PS: Clinical Handbook of Psychiatry and the Law, 3rd Edition. Philadelphia, PA, Lippincott Williams & Wilkins, 2000

Kapp MB: Decisional capacity in theory and practice: legal process versus 'bumbling through.' Aging Ment Health 6(4):413–417, 2002 12425775

Karlawish J: Measuring decision-making capacity in cognitively impaired individuals. Neurosignals 16(1):91–98, 2008 18097164

Karlawish JHT, Casarett D, Propert KJ, et al: Relationship between Alzheimer's disease severity and patient participation in decisions about their medical care. J Geriatr Psychiatry Neurol 15(2):68–72, 2002 12083595

Kim SY, Karlawish JH, Caine ED: Current state of research on decision-making competence of cognitively impaired elderly persons. Am J Geriatr Psychiatry 10(2):151–165, 2002 11925276

Moye J, Butz SW, Marson DC, et al: A conceptual model and assessment template for capacity evaluation in adult guardianship. Gerontologist 47(5):591–603, 2007 17989401

Nuffield Council on Bioethics: Dementia: Ethical Issues. London, Nuffield Council on Bioethics, 2009. Available at: http://nuffieldbioethics.org/wp-content/uploads/2014/07/Dementia-report-Oct-09.pdf. Accessed August 19, 2018.

Palmer BW, Harmell AL: Assessment of healthcare decision-making capacity. Arch Clin Neuropsychol 31(6):530–540, 2016 27551024

Rissmiller DJ, Musser E, Rhoades W, et al: A survey of use of a durable power of attorney to admit geropsychiatric patients. Psychiatr Serv 52(1):98–100, 2001 11141537

Roberts LW: Informed consent and the capacity for voluntarism. Am J Psychiatry 159(5):705–712, 2002 11986120

Roberts LW, Dyer AR (eds): Ethics in Mental Health Care (Concise Guides Series; Hales RE, ed). Arlington, VA, American Psychiatric Publishing, 2004

Treloar A, Crugel M, Prasanna A, et al: Ethical dilemmas: should antipsychotics ever be prescribed for people with dementia? Br J Psychiatry 197(2):88–90, 2010 20679257

Walaszek A: Clinical ethics issues in geriatric psychiatry. Psychiatr Clin North Am 32(2):343–359, 2009 19486818

Walaszek A: Ethical issues in the care of individuals with dementia, in Dementia. Edited by McNamara P. Santa Barbara, CA, ABC-CLIO, 2011, pp 123–150

Yaffe MJ, Wolfson C, Lithwick M, et al: Development and validation of a tool to improve physician identification of elder abuse: the Elder Abuse Suspicion Index (EASI). J Elder Abuse Negl 20(3):276–300, 2008 18928055

APPENDIX

Pre-evaluation Form

PRE-EVALUATION FORM

Please complete this form and bring it with you to your appointment. If you cannot complete this form, please ask a family member to do so.

Name: _____

Date of birth: ___ / ___ / _____

Best phone number to reach you: _____

Please list up to 3 relatives you would like to be involved in your care.

Name: _____ Relationship: _____

Phone number: _____

Name: _____ Relationship: _____

Phone number: _____

Name: _____ Relationship: _____

Phone number: _____

Please list your Health Care Power of Attorney, if you have one.

Name: _____ Phone: _____

Please list all the doctors currently involved in your care, starting with your primary care doctor.

Name: _____

Clinic: _____

Phone number: _____

Name: _____

Clinic: _____

Phone number: _____

Name: _____

Clinic: _____

Phone number: _____

Name: _____

Clinic: _____

Phone number: _____

Pharmacy name: _____

Pharmacy phone number: _____

Your Name: _____

Please list your current medications, including any over-the-counter remedies, vitamins, and herbal products. Include the reason why you are taking each medication.

Medication	Dose	Schedule	Reason

If you run out of room, please use the other side of the page.

List any medications you are allergic to, and what reactions you have had:

_____

Please check any medical conditions you have:

- ☐ arthritis
- ☐ high blood pressure
- ☐ high cholesterol
- ☐ heart attack or angina
- ☐ congestive heart failure
- ☐ emphysema (COPD)
- ☐ diabetes
- ☐ heartburn or reflux disease
- ☐ glaucoma
- ☐ hearing loss
- ☐ cancer – if so, list what kind:
- ☐ other – list:

- ☐ chronic pain
- ☐ thyroid disease
- ☐ head injury or concussion
- ☐ stroke or TIA
- ☐ Alzheimer's disease
- ☐ Parkinson's disease
- ☐ osteoporosis
- ☐ sleep apnea
- ☐ cataracts
- ☐ problems with balance

_____

Please check any other health concerns you have had in the last month:

- ☐ weight loss
- ☐ change in appetite
- ☐ problems sleeping
- ☐ can't concentrate
- ☐ poor memory
- ☐ trouble finding words
- ☐ sadness or depression
- ☐ worrying or anxiety
- ☐ irritability
- ☐ shakiness or tremor
- ☐ frequent urination
- ☐ changes in vision

- ☐ weakness
- ☐ get tired or fatigued easily
- ☐ dizziness
- ☐ headaches
- ☐ chest pain
- ☐ short of breath
- ☐ abdominal pain
- ☐ nausea or vomiting
- ☐ diarrhea
- ☐ constipation
- ☐ fever
- ☐ rash

Your Name: _____

For each of the activities below, please check the appropriate box:

	I can do this myself	I need help doing this, but have adequate help	I need help doing this, and do not have adequate help
Driving	☐	☐	☐
Paying my bills	☐	☐	☐
Housekeeping	☐	☐	☐
Making my meals	☐	☐	☐
Grocery shopping	☐	☐	☐
Using the phone	☐	☐	☐
Taking my medications	☐	☐	☐
Feeding myself	☐	☐	☐
Getting to the rest room in time	☐	☐	☐
Walking	☐	☐	☐
Getting dressed in the morning	☐	☐	☐
Bathing regularly	☐	☐	☐

Please indicate if you use or have used any of the following substances:

tobacco	☐ past	☐ current	amount:
alcohol	☐ past	☐ current	amount:
marijuana	☐ past	☐ current	amount:
narcotics	☐ past	☐ current	amount:

Do you have any firearms at home?

    ☐ no
    ☐ yes   ⟶   ☐ one or more guns is loaded
                   ☐ one or more guns is unlocked

Do you have any concerns about the following?

    ☐ falling, or nearly falling down
    ☐ getting lost driving
    ☐ getting into accidents driving, or near accidents
    ☐ someone is taking advantage of me or stealing from me
    ☐ someone is hurting me, or trying to hurt me
    ☐ trouble taking my medications correctly
    ☐ trouble making decisions
    ☐ pain that is not well controlled
    ☐ my family members are stressed
    ☐ not getting the help I need at home
    ☐ planning for the future

What specific concerns would you like to have addressed during your visit?

Index

Page numbers printed in **boldface** type refer to tables or figures.